ONE WEEK LOAN

Renew Books on PHONE-it: 01443 654456

Books are to be returned on or before the last date below

Treforest Learning Resources Centre
University of Glamorgan CF37 1DL

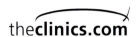

CLINICS IN SPORTS MEDICINE

Sports Injury Outcomes and Prevention

GUEST EDITOR
Joseph M. Hart, PhD, ATC

CONSULTING EDITOR
Mark D. Miller, MD

July 2008 • Volume 27 • Number 3

SAUNDERS

An Imprint of Elsevier, Inc.
PHILADELPHIA   LONDON   TORONTO   MONTREAL   SYDNEY   TOKYO

W.B. SAUNDERS COMPANY
A Division of Elsevier Inc.

1600 John F. Kennedy Blvd. • Suite 1800 • Philadelphia, Pennsylvania 19103

http://www.theclinics.com

CLINICS IN SPORTS MEDICINE
July 2008
Editor: Debora Dellapena

Volume 27, Number 3
ISSN 0278-5919
ISBN-13: 978-1-4160-6354-4
ISBN-10: 1-4160-6354-4

The ideas and opinions expressed in *Clinics in Sports Medicine* do not necessarily reflect those of the Publisher. The Publisher does not assume any responsibility for any injury and/or damage to persons or property arising out of or related to any use of the material contained in this periodical. The reader is advised to check the appropriate medical literature and the product information currently provided by the manufacturer of each drug to be administered to verify the dosage, the method and duration of administration, or contraindications. It is the responsibility of the treating physician or other health care professional, relying on independent experience and knowledge of the patient, to determine drug dosages and the best treatment for the patient. Mention of any product in this issue should not be construed as endorsement by the contributors, editors, or the Publisher of the product or manufacturers' claims.

Clinics in Sports Medicine (ISSN 0278-5919) is published quarterly by Elsevier Inc., 360 Park Avenue South, New York, NY 10010-1710. Months of publication are January, April, July, and October. Business and Editorial Offices: 1600 John F. Kennedy Blvd., Suite 1800, Philadelphia, PA 19103-2899. Customer Service Offices: 6277 Sea Harbor Drive, Orlando, FL 32887-4800. Periodicals postage paid at New York, NY, and additional mailing offices. Subscription prices are $230.00 per year (US individuals), $357.00 per year (US institutions), $115.00 per year (US students), $260.00 per year (Canadian individuals), $423.00 per year (Canadian institutions), $151.00 (Canadian students), $297.00 per year (foreign individuals), $423.00 per year (foreign institutions), and $151.00 per year (foreign students). Foreign air speed delivery is included in all *Clinics* subscription prices. All prices are subject to change without notice. POSTMASTER: Send address changes to *Clinics in Sports Medicine*, Elsevier Periodicals Customer Service, 6277 Sea Harbor Drive, Orlando, FL 32887-4800. Customer Service: 1-800-654-2452 (US). From outside the United States, call 1-407-563-6020. Fax: 1-407-363-9661. E-mail: JournalsCustomerService-usa@elsevier.com.

Clinics in Sports Medicine is covered in *Index Medicus, Current Contents/Clinical Medicine, Excerpta Medica,* and *ISI/Biomed.*

Printed in the United States of America.

ELSEVIER
SAUNDERS

CLINICS IN SPORTS MEDICINE

Sports Injury Outcomes and Prevention

CONSULTING EDITOR

MARK D. MILLER, MD, Professor, Department of Orthopaedic Surgery; Director, Division of Sports Medicine, University of Virginia Health System, Charlottesville, Virginia

GUEST EDITOR

JOSEPH M. HART, PhD, ATC, Assistant Professor of Research, Department of Orthopaedic Surgery, University of Virginia, Charlottesville, Virginia

CONTRIBUTORS

JAMES R. BEAZELL, PT, DPT, OCS, FAAOMPT, ATC, Clinical Coordinator, University of Virginia-Healthsouth, Charlottesville, Virginia

JENSEN L. BRENT, BS, CSCS, Sports Medicine Biodynamics Center and Human Performance Laboratory Cincinnati Children's Hospital Medical Center, Cincinnati Children's Hospital, Cincinnati, Ohio

DONALD A. CHU, PhD, PT, ATC, CSCS, Professor, Graduate Program in Athletic Training, Rocky Mountain University of Health Professions, Provo, Utah; Clinic Director, Athercare Fitness and Rehabilitation Clinic, Alameda; Professor, Ohlone College, Newark, California

CRAIG R. DENEGAR, PT, PhD, ATC, Professor; Department Head, Department of Physical Therapy, Neag School of Education, University of Connecticut, Storrs, Connecticut

TODD A. EVANS, PhD, ATC, LAT, Associate Professor; Division Chair, Division of Athletic Training, Human Performance Center, University of Northern Iowa, Cedar Falls, Iowa

JULIE FRITZ, PhD, PT, ATC, The University of Utah, College of Health, Salt Lake City, Utah

TERRY L. GRINDSTAFF, DPT, ATC, Assistant Athletic Trainer, Department of Athletics; Doctoral Fellow, Exercise and Sport Injury Laboratory, University of Virginia, Charlottesville, Virginia

ROBERT R. HAMMILL, MA, ATC, Assistant Professor, Health and Exercise Science, Bridgewater College, Bridgewater, Virginia

JOSEPH M. HART, PhD, ATC, Assistant Professor of Research, Department of Orthopaedic Surgery, University of Virginia, Charlottesville, Virginia

JEFFREY HEBERT, DC, Department of Physical Therapy, The University of Utah, College of Health, Salt Lake City, Utah

JAY HERTEL, PhD, ATC, Associate Professor of Kinesiology, Department of Human Services, University of Virginia, Exercise and Sport Injury Lab, Charlottesville, Virginia

TIMOTHY E. HEWETT, PhD, FACSM, Sports Medicine Biodynamics Center and Human Performance Laboratory Cincinnati Children's Hospital Medical Center, Cincinnati Children's Hospital; Department of Pediatrics, Orthopaedic Surgery, College of Medicine and the Departments of Biomedical Engineering and Rehabilitation Sciences, University of Cincinnati, Cincinnati, Ohio

CHRISTOPHER D. INGERSOLL, PhD, ATC, Joe H. Gieck Professor of Sports Medicine; Chair, Department of Human Services; Director, Exercise and Sport Injury Laboratory, University of Virginia, Charlottesville, Virginia

SHANE KOPPENHAVER, MPT, The University of Utah, College of Health, Salt Lake City, Utah

CARL G. MATTACOLA, PhD, ATC, Associate Professor; Director, Division of Athletic Training, University of Kentucky, College of Health Sciences, Lexington, Kentucky

PATRICK O. MCKEON, PhD, ATC, CSCS, Assistant Professor, Division of Athletic Training, University of Kentucky, College of Health Sciences, Lexington, Kentucky

LORI A. MICHENER, PhD, PT, ATC, SCS, Associate Professor, Department of Physical Therapy, Virginia Commonwealth University, Medical College of Virginia Campus, Richmond, Virginia

GREGORY D. MYER, MS, CSCS, Sports Medicine Biodynamics Center and Human Performance Laboratory Cincinnati Children's Hospital Medical Center, Cincinnati Children's Hospital, Cincinnati, Ohio; Graduate Program in Athletic Training, Rocky Mountain University of Health Professions, Provo, Utah

JOSEPH B. MYERS, PhD, ATC, University of North Carolina at Chapel Hill, Department of Exercise and Sport Science, Chapel Hill, North Carolina

SAKIKO OYAMA, MS, ATC, University of North Carolina at Chapel Hill, Department of Exercise and Sport Science, Chapel Hill, North Carolina

RIANN M. PALMIERI-SMITH, PhD, ATC, Assistant Professor, Athletic Training, Movement Science, and Orthopaedics, Division of Kinesiology; Department of Orthopaedic Surgery; Bone and Joint Injury Prevention and Rehabilitation Center, University of Michigan, Ann Arbor, Michigan

ERIC PARENT, PhD, PT, Department of Physical Therapy, The University of Alberta, Faculty of Rehabilitation Medicine, Edmonton, Canada

BRIAN G. PIETROSIMONE, MEd, ATC, Doctoral Fellow, Exercise and Sport Injury Laboratory, University of Virginia, Charlottesville, Virginia

ALISON R. SNYDER, PhD, ATC, Assistant Professor, Department of Interdisciplinary Health Sciences, Athletic Training Program, A.T. Still University, Mesa, Arizona

ABBEY C. THOMAS, MEd, ATC, Division of Kinesiology, University of Michigan, Ann Arbor, Michigan

BRADY L. TRIPP, PhD, ATC, Coordinator, Post-Professional Athletic Training Education Program; Director, Golf Academy and Sport Biomechanics Laboratory; Assistant Professor, Department of Athletic Training, College of Nursing and Health Sciences, Florida International University, Miami, Florida

LUZITA I. VELA, PhD, ATC, LAT, Assistant Professor and Clinical Coordinator of Athletic Training Education, Department of Health, Physical Education and Recreation, Texas State University, San Marcos, Texas

EDWARD M. WOJTYS, MD, Professor, Department of Orthopaedic Surgery; Bone and Joint Injury Prevention and Rehabilitation Center, University of Michigan, Ann Arbor, Michigan

ELSEVIER
SAUNDERS

CLINICS IN SPORTS MEDICINE

Sports Injury Outcomes and Prevention

CONTENTS VOLUME 27 • NUMBER 3 • JULY 2008

> Clear and directed outcomes assessment is an integral part of clinical decision making. For sports medicine clinicians, it is crucial to choose appropriate instruments that are grounded in disablement theory, designed to measure the ability of a physically active population, and have established psychometric properties. Although there is no instrument ideal for every situation in sports medicine, there are important guidelines that a clinician can follow that will allow for the selection of an appropriate instrument. The purposes of this article are to (1) introduce the reader to self-report instruments available, with particular attention to those most appropriate for athletic populations, (2) describe the relationship between disablement paradigms and health-related self-report instruments, and (3) describe the process of instrument development.

Ankle Injury Outcomes and Prevention

> The presence of sensorimotor deficits in patients who have suffered ankle sprains or who have chronic ankle instability has been recognized for several decades; however, a body of research literature has developed that elucidates potential physiologic explanations for these deficits. Alterations in a spectrum of sensorimotor measures make it apparent that conscious perception of afferent somatosensory information, reflex responses, and efferent motor control deficits are present with ankle instability. The specific origin of these deficits local to the ankle ligaments or at the spinal or supraspinal levels of motor control have yet to be fully elucidated. It is clear, however, that both feedback and feedforward mechanisms of motor control are altered with ankle instability.

The uses of external support and balance/coordination training have demonstrated to be effective interventions for the prevention of ankle sprains, especially in those who have a history of ankle sprain. The purpose of this article is to identify areas where evidence has been established to support the use of these interventions for the prevention and enhancement of outcomes of lateral ankle sprain. In addition, areas of deficiency in the evidence are discussed related to these interventions. Finally, future directions for clinicians and researchers as per the use of these interventions are discussed.

The neuromuscular consequences of anterior cruciate ligament (ACL) injury are important considerations because these deficits play a crucial role in a patient's recovery following ACL injury or reconstruction. The purpose of this article is to review and synthesize the known neuromuscular consequences of ACL injury and reconstruction. Specifically, changes in somatosensation, muscle activation, muscle strength, atrophy, balance, biomechanics, and patient-oriented outcomes are discussed. Understanding neuromuscular consequences aids in the construction of optimized rehabilitation strategies.

The primary objectives of ACL surgery and rehabilitation are to restore knee function to preinjury levels and promote long-term joint health. Often these goals are not achieved, however. The quadriceps is critical to dynamic joint stability, and weakness of this muscle group is related to poor functional outcomes. Because of this, identifying strategies to minimize quadriceps weakness following ACL injury and reconstruction is of great clinical interest. This article reviews the current literature and critically discusses current rehabilitation approaches to restore quadriceps muscle function after ACL reconstruction.

This article provide evidences to outline a novel theory used to define the mechanisms related to increased risk of ACL injury in female athletes. In addition, this discussion will include theoretical constructs for the description of the mechanisms that lead to increased risk. Finally, a clinical application section will outline novel neuromuscular training techniques designed to target deficits that underlie the proposed mechanism of increased risk of knee injury in female athletes.

Low Back Pain Outcomes and Prevention

Recurring episodes of low back pain present a dilemma for patients and clinicians. Patients who experience disability caused by repeated low back pain episodes are limited in their activities of daily living and may experience inappropriate neuromuscular adaptations to maintain and/or preserve function. Unfortunately, it is likely that these changes create an environment where lower extremity and spine joints are exposed to unusual and possibly excessive forces while attenuating impact from walking, running, or other activities. Individuals who want to maintain a healthy lifestyle may be restricted because of recurring and disabling nonspecific low back pain. Individuals who must continue with normal and necessary activities of daily living may choose an adaptive mechanism to preserve functional gait. Some individuals may use an adaptive strategy that is unfavorable, possibly exposing muscles and joints to further injury or long-term degenerative processes.

Treatment-based classification, one approach to subgrouping patients with "nonspecific" lower back pain, focuses on identifying clusters of findings from the history and clinical examination that predict a more favorable outcome with a specific treatment approach. By matching patients with the appropriate specific exercise, stabilization exercise, spinal manipulation, or traction treatment, providers may expect a high probability of a successful clinical outcome. This article reviews the evidence for various interventions commonly used in the treatment of lower back pain.

Shoulder Injury Outcomes and Prevention

When the shoulder is subjected to an injurious mechanism, a cascade of effects results. These effects include tissue pathology and the manifestation of pain. Sensorimotor alterations also manifest, most likely as a result of tissue pathology and pain. The combination of the tissue pathology, pain, and sensorimotor alterations all directly affect outcome following injury, and thus need to be addressed by the clinician treating the shoulder injury to fully restore function. This article discusses how the sensorimotor system contributes to shoulder function and how it is altered with shoulder injury, thereby affecting outcome.

This article provides an understanding of patient-based shoulder outcome tools and the conceptual framework of disablement models from which the patient-based outcome tools are based. To allow for the evaluation of function, disability, and health-related quality of life in patients suffering from shoulder pain and in particular those whose shoulders have high physical demands, the use of shoulder self-report patient-oriented outcome tools must become standard of practice. A wide variety of available outcome tools demonstrate acceptable levels of measurement properties and are appropriate for virtually every patient with a shoulder disorder.

This article reviews the basic principles of restoring sensorimotor (SMS) function and evidence-based outcome assessments and describes their integration into treating patients who have shoulder dysfunction. When integrated clinically, the principles of restoring SMS function act in synergy with those of functional outcome-based practices.

ELSEVIER
SAUNDERS

CLINICS IN SPORTS MEDICINE

Clin Sports Med 27 (2008) xiii

CLINICS IN SPORTS MEDICINE

Foreword

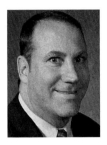

Mark D. Miller, MD
Consulting Editor

I t is my sincere pleasure to introduce this issue of *Clinics in Sports Medicine* dedicated to outcomes and prevention of sports injuries with particular focus on neuromuscular issues and evidence-based treatment. Dr. Joe Hart, who has extensive experience in this area, has put together an all-star team in this issue. All aspects of this important topic are addressed, beginning with outcome measurements and including ankle, knee, shoulder, and spine neuromuscular considerations.

The issue is organized into five major areas: ankle, knee, low back and shoulder, where articles present neuromuscular and subjective outcomes, following injury and evidence-based recommendations for prevention of injury and re-injury. Team physicians, athletic trainers, and other rehabilitation specialists should be well informed about contemporary theory and issues pertaining to injury outcomes in active individuals and athletes. A comprehensive approach to treating injuries in an active population is essential to improving function and preventing further injury as the injured athlete returns to his/her sport of choice. All members of the sports medicine team will certainly benefit from this thorough review of outcomes and treatment for sports-related joint injuries.

Mark D. Miller, MD
Department of Orthopaedic Surgery
Division of Sports Medicine
University of Virginia Health System
P.O. Box 800753
UVA Dept of Orthopaedic Surgery
Charlottesville, VA 22908-0159, USA

E-mail address: mdm3p@virginia.edu

0278-5919/08/$ – see front matter
doi:10.1016/j.csm.2008.03.007

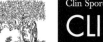

Clin Sports Med 27 (2008) xv

CLINICS IN SPORTS MEDICINE

Preface

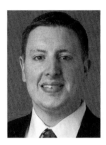

Joseph M. Hart, PhD, ATC

This issue of *Clinics in Sports Medicine* is devoted to outcomes and prevention of sports-related injuries. Developing the most effective treatment strategies for restoring normal neuromuscular function following major joint injury requires an understanding of outcomes following injury, including deficits in neuromuscular function. Through research and evidence-based practice, clinicians and scholars derive facts and develop theories with a common goal of enhancing the quality of life for injured individuals. This is common ground for researchers and clinicians: identifying the problem or injury through an interview and controlled testing, thereby prescribing the most suitable treatment.

In this issue, an introductory article describing instruments used in the field of sports medicine to assess sports-related injury outcomes provides an essential framework and starting point. Each section (ankle, knee, low back, and shoulder) contains a series of articles that reviews specific sports injury outcomes, followed by articles devoted to current and evidence-based treatment strategies aimed at restoring normal neuromuscular and musculoskeletal function.

I am truly appreciative to the authors who have contributed to this issue of *Clinics in Sports Medicine*. Together, we have assembled an excellent review of outcomes following orthopaedic injury in an active population, as well as treatment strategies to prevent injury and promote optimal outcomes in injured persons.

Joseph M. Hart, PhD, ATC
Department of Orthopaedic Surgery
University of Virginia
PO Box 800159
Charlottesville, VA 22908

E-mail address: joehart@virginia.edu

0278-5919/08/$ – see front matter
doi:10.1016/j.csm.2008.03.003

Clin Sports Med 27 (2008) 339–351

CLINICS IN SPORTS MEDICINE

ELSEVIER
SAUNDERS

Evidence-Based Sports Medicine: Outcomes Instruments for Active Populations

Craig R. Denegar, PT, PhD, ATC[a],*,
Luzita I. Vela, PhD, ATC, LAT[b],
Todd A. Evans, PhD, ATC, LAT[c]

[a]Department of Physical Therapy, Neag School of Education, University of Connecticut,
Koons Hall–101A, 358 Mansfield Road, U-2101, Storrs, CT 06269-2064, USA
[b]Department of Health, Physical Education and Recreation, Texas State University,
A 126 Jowers, San Marcos, TX 78666, USA
[c]Division of Athletic Training, Human Performance Center, University of Northern Iowa,
2351 Hudson Road, Cedar Falls, IA 50614-0244, USA

Sackett and colleagues [1] defined evidence-based medicine as "the integration of best research evidence with clinical expertise and patient values." Evidence related to patient care may inform the evaluative or diagnostic process and the prescription of preventative or therapeutic interventions, or describe the progression of disease processes. This issue of *Clinics in Sports Medicine* is devoted to the latter two subjects, with articles describing the sequelae of sports-related injury including ankle, shoulder, knee, and low back, coupled with reports that address treatments and treatment responses.

The data that constitute the evidence related to disease progression and treatment efficacy can be categorized in various ways. Data, for example, may be categorized based on a disablement paradigm to include measures of impairment, functional limitation, disability, and quality of life. Disablement paradigms are useful in understanding the sequence of problems and limitations that occur after an injury. They also create a theoretic framework with associated constructs that clinicians use to measure and document outcomes. There are numerous paradigms used in sports medicine created by the World Health Organization (WHO), Institute of Medicine (IOM) and National Center for Medical Rehabilitation Research (NCMRR). Most of these paradigms evolved from the work completed by Saad Nagi, the social scientist, who described the disablement process in the 1960s. A description of the common measurement constructs will be included in this article.

Data also can be categorized based on the method by which it is acquired. Clinician-collected data in cases of musculoskeletal conditions can include

*Corresponding author. *E-mail address:* craig.denegar@uconn.edu (C.R. Denegar).

0278-5919/08/$ – see front matter
doi:10.1016/j.csm.2008.02.002

measures such as strength, range of motion, or performance during functional tasks (eg, running, hopping, jumping). Although useful in planning the care of individual patients, following the course of diseases, and comparing treatment efficacy, measurements obtained by a clinician do not span the elements of disablement paradigms. Comprehensive assessment of disablement requires inclusion of patient self-report of the impact of his or her condition on the ability to perform tasks normal to daily life on quality of life. This article's purposes are to:

- Introduce the reader to self-report instruments available, with particular attention to those most appropriate for athletic populations
- Describe the relationship between disablement paradigms and health-related self-report instruments
- Describe the process of instrument development

There are various self-report instruments available to clinicians. The challenge, however, is to select the instruments that best meet the needs of the clinician or patient or best answer the questions posed in clinical research. Self-report instruments can be classified as general health, condition-specific, or region- specific. Examples of each are listed in Table 1.

This patient self-reports list is not an exhaustive posting but does illustrate the number of options from which the clinician or researcher can choose. This listing also is not intended to convey that these instruments perform well in a particular circumstance or have been evaluated fully with contemporary research methods. In fact, none have been validated in a solely athletic population, and there is much work to be done in this area before such applications can be made with confidence of valid data. This said, these instruments likely provide the best opportunities to inform decisions regarding treatment. The selection of an instrument can be challenging. Careful review may be necessary to select an instrument that best measures what the clinician or researcher sets out to measure and ensure the instrument performs well within the context (setting and population sampled) in which assessment occurs. The development of self-report instruments is an emerging science. An understanding of how self-report instruments are developed and the desirable psychometric properties for self-report instruments will assist in the assessment of new instruments and the instrument selection process.

DISABLEMENT PARADIGMS: CONSTRUCTS AND CONCEPTS

Disablement is the sequence of interrelated but discrete events that take place as a result of pathology, and ultimately it leads to disability or participation restrictions. Multiple organizations have described the disablement process identifying similar constructs while using differing terminology [2–7]. Fig. 1 demonstrates the constructs used to describe the disablement process, beginning on the left of the figure with the source that begins the disablement process, continuing on to the effects at the local, person and social levels. Under each construct are terms used by the differing paradigms to describe the problems associated with disablement at the respective level. For example, a common term used to describe a problem at the local level during the disablement process is impairment. Under the paradigm are two additional constructs typically included in disablement models but not parts of the main pathway. Mediators of the disablement process include individual differences and environmental factors and are considered contextual factors. Lastly, quality of life (QOL) has a bidirectional effect on the disablement process, indicating that changes in QOL can enhance or detract from the disablement process. Additionally, the disablement process affects QOL.

The paradigms were created for numerous reasons: (1) to understand the full disablement experience, (2) to create constructs that could be defined and measured, and (3) to elucidate the relationships along the disablement pathway. Much of what is understood about disablement comes from the work completed by Saad Nagi. Nagi's influences still can be seen in all of the evolved paradigms [3]. The original disablement frameworks provided by the WHO, IOM, and NCMRR used terminology such as disability and handicap. Over time, some paradigms deleted the use of these words because of their negative connotations [8]. Despite their differences, all three models have focused on the importance of recognizing the disablement process as a patient-centered process in which expectations and environment play a major role in how a patient responds to interventions and progresses through the disablement process.

The importance of creating a theoretic framework such as disablement paradigms is to ensure a common language for clinical outcomes. Some confusion may exist because of the differing terminology used in the various paradigms. In fact, a general trend in the rehabilitation sciences is to move toward adopting a specific paradigm for the field to avoid such confusion. For example, physical therapists developed the *Guide to Physical Therapist Practice* in the 1990s using terminology based on Nagi's work [9]. Additionally, other fields have used the models created by the NCMRR, WHO, and IOM. The purpose of this section is to distill the overarching concepts across all disablement paradigms as they apply to outcomes assessment and to focus on the strengths of the paradigms.

Inherent in all disablement paradigms is the theory that pathology, such as a musculoskeletal injury, will have local effects that potentially can lead to systemic problems. Stated simply, the models recognize that injury affects a patient at the organ, person, and societal levels [8]. For example, disablement paradigms assert that following an injury the patient will complain of impairments that are localized to the area of injury. Examples include pain, decreased range of motion, strength loss, and instability. Localized impairments then can lead to restrictions in normal function that tend to limit basic actions that patients may perform daily such as sitting, squatting, reaching, bending, and turning. Sport-related examples include running, jumping, throwing, turning, and cutting. At this point in the paradigm, one sees that a localized pathology can start to affect the patient globally. Function restrictions in turn lead to disability or participation restrictions that are defined as the inability to complete normal activities that a patient would chose to complete in a sociocultural and physical

Table 1
Self-report outcomes instruments for musculoskeletal injuries

General health
Short Form 36 (SF- 36)	Ware JE, Jr., Sherbourne CD. The MOS 36-item short form health survey (SF-36). I. Conceptual framework and item selection. Med Care 1992; 30(6):473–83.
Short Form 12 (SF-12)	Ware J, Jr, Kosinski M, Keller SD. A 12-item short-form health survey: construction of scales and preliminary tests of reliability and validity. Med Care 1996;34(3):220–33.
Musculoskeletal Function Assessment (MFA)	Martin DP, Engelberg R, Agel J, et al. Development of a musculoskeletal extremity health status instrument: the musculoskeletal function assessment instrument. J Orthop Res 1996; 14(2):173–81.
Short Musculoskeletal Function Assessment (SMFA)	Swiontkowski MF, Engelberg R, Martin DP, Agel J. Short musculoskeletal function assessment questionnaire: validity, reliability, and responsiveness. J Bone Joint Surg Am 1999;81(9):1245–60.

Low back
Oswestry Disability Index	Fairbank JCT, Couper J, Davies JB. The Oswestry low back pain questionnaire. Physiotherapy 1980;66:271–3.
Roland Morris Low Back Pain Questionnaire	Roland M, Morris R. A study of the natural history of back pain. Part 1: development of a reliable and sensitive measure of disability in low back pain. Spine 1983;8:141–4.

Knee
Knee Injury and Osteoarthritis Outcome Score (KOOS)	Roos EM, Roos HP, Lohmander LS et al. Knee injury and osteoarthritis outcome score (KOOS): development of a self-administered outcomes measure J Orthop Sports Phys Ther 1998; 28:88–96.
Western Ontario and McMaster Universities Osteoarthritis Index (WOMAC)	Bellamy N, Buchanan WW, Goldsmith CH, et al. Validation study of WOMAC: a health status instrument for measuring clinically important patient relevant outcomes to antirheumatic drug therapy in patients with osteoarthritis of the hip or knee. J Rheumatol 1988;15:1833–40.
Cincinnati Knee Rating System	Noyes FR, Barber SD, Mooar LA. A rationale for assessing sports activity levels and limitations in knee disorders. Clin Orthop 1989;246:238–49.
Kujala Patellofemoral Score (AKPS)	Kujala UM, Jaakkola LH, Koskinen SK. Scoring of patellofemoral disorders. Arthroscopy 1993; 9:159–63.
International Knee Documentation Committee Knee Scoring System (IKDC)	Hefti F, Muller W, Jakob RP, et al. Evaluation of knee ligament injuries with the IKDC form. Knee Surg Sports Traumatol Arthrosc 1993;1:226–34.

(continued on next page)

Table 1
(continued)

Foot and ankle	
Foot and Ankle Ability Measure (FAAM)	Martin RL, Irrgang JJ, Burdett RG, et al. Evidence of validity for the Foot and Ankle Ability Measure (FAAM) Foot Ankle Int 2005;26(11):968–83.
Lower Extremity Functional Scale (LEFS)	Binkley JM, Stratford PW, Lott SA, et al. The Lower Extremity Functional Scale (LEFS): scale development, measurement properties, and clinical application. North American Orthopaedic Rehabilitation Research Network. Phys Ther 1999;79(4):371–83.
Victorian Institute of Sport Assessment-Achilles Questionnaire (VISA-A)	Robinson JM, Cook JL, Purdam C, et al. The VISA-A questionnaire: a valid and reliable index of the clinical severity of Achilles tendinopathy Br J Sports Med 2001;35(5):335–41.
Shoulder and upper extremity	
Disabilities of the Arm, Shoulder and Hand (DASH)	Hudak PL, Amadio PC, Bombardier C. The Upper Extremity Collaborative Group (UECG). Development of an upper extremity outcome measure: the DASH (Disabilities of the Arm, Shoulder and Hand) [corrected]. Am J Ind Med 1996;29:602–8.
Western Ontario Rotator Cuff Index (WORC)	Kirkley A, Alvarez C, Griffin S. The development and evaluation of a disease-specific quality-of-life questionnaire for disorders of the rotator cuff: The Western Ontario Rotator Cuff Index. Clin J Sport Med 2003;13(2):84–92.
Cervical spine	
Cervical Spine Outcomes Questionnaire	BenDebba M, Heller J, Ducker TB, Eisinger JM. Cervical Spine Outcomes Questionnaire: its development and psychometric properties. Spine 2002;27(19):2116–23.

Available patient self-report instruments by classification. One reference related to development and psychometric performance is provided for each.

environment [3]. Like its predecessor, disability can affect a patient within the sports realm and in activities of daily living. The important distinction between functional limitations and disability is that function is defined by actions, while disability is defined by activities [6]. In addition, disability is a social experience that is influenced by the patient's environment [10].

Throughout any point along the disablement paradigm, QOL may be affected adversely by an injury. QOL is a broad conceptualization that encompasses general and mental health perceptions in addition to physical, social, and role functioning [10,11]. The inclusion of QOL assessment in clinical studies has gained tremendous popularity over the past 20 years as an important indicator of success [12,13]. Now generic outcomes assessment that includes disablement and QOL are referred to health-related QOL (HRQOL) tools. McAllister and colleagues [14] found that elite athletes scored higher on HRQOL measurements

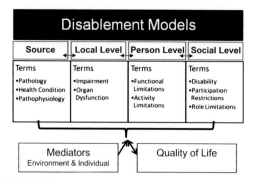

Fig. 1. Disablement models and terminology (*Data from* Nagi S. Disability concepts revisited: implications for prevention. In: Pope A, Tarlov A, editors. Disability in America: toward a national agenda for prevention. Washington, DC: National Academy Press; 1991. p. 309–27. Brandt E, Pope A. Enabling America: assessing the role of rehabilitation science and engineering. Washington, DC: National Academy Press; 1997. International classification of functioning, disability and health. Geneva (IL): World Health Organization; 2001. Whiteneck G. Conceptual models of disability: past, present, and future. In: Field M, Jette A, Martin L, editors. Workshop on disability in America: a new look–summary and background papers. National Acadamies Press; 2006. Accessed June 10, 2006).

when compared with a sedentary population, indicating that QOL measurement is particularly important in elite athletes. Furthermore, the researchers found that following injury, all QOL domains, including mental health, social function, vitality, and general health were affected negatively. The results of this study indicate that QOL is affected greatly after injury and warrants measurement to fully assess the clinical effectiveness of an intervention.

Note that all of the disablement paradigms use a linear model to describe the complex interactions between and among the disablement constructs. In actuality, the relationships between the constructs are recursive in nature, indicating that the relationships are not unidirectional but cyclical [6]. This concept emphasizes the intricate nature of disablement and demonstrates the importance of two factors that aid or hinder the disablement process: context and expectations.

Context and Expectations

Disability is an innately personal concept that centers on a patient's expectations for health, QOL, and inclusion. In fact, disability level is predicated highly on the desires of the patient. This does not mean that disability is purely about patient satisfaction. Rather, disability is the gap between a person's capabilities and expectations, signifying that patient values are an important part of the disablement process. This is particularly important concept in sports medicine for several reasons. Typically patients who participate in sport have much higher expectations for function when compared with a sedentary population. In addition, the physical demands of sport require outcomes that allow a patient to place greater demands on the musculoskeletal system. Furthermore, because disability is a patient-centered experience, self-reports of function, disability and quality of life are important outcomes to measure. This means that a clinician must progress beyond objective, clinician-centered tests such as impairment to truly understand the effects of disability on a patient.

Many researchers have asserted that the disabling process can be stopped or avoided given the patient–environment interaction [4,5,8,15]. Since their creation, disablement paradigms have focused on the importance of creating external support systems to limit the effects of disability on a patient. This said, context plays a big role in the disabling process. For example, a patient who has impairment, such as limited knee range of motion, may not have limitations in accessing a second story room if he or she has access to a ramp or similar support. A sport-related example is limiting painful knee hyperextension by bracing a patient during activity. Clinicians must understand that the context of injury, treatment, surgery, and rehabilitations all play a role in patient outcomes and may account for why similar patients who have the same injury may report considerably differing outcomes.

Applications for Measurement

Although disablement is a theory, the paradigms can be applied directly in measuring outcomes. The basic premise behind much of disablement research focuses on the inclusion of all the disablement constructs when measuring and documenting outcomes. Because disablement paradigms place importance on various levels of functioning (physical, mental and social), they help to frame the clinical outcomes that are important and truly indicative of meaningful change over time. Furthermore, both clinician-report and patient-report assessments are warranted following injury.

An examination of the literature illustrates that impairments are the most commonly researched and documented type of data within sports medicine; yet research has shown that impairments alone do not disclose the nature and severity of disability fully. This indicates that researchers and clinicians should look beyond simple impairment measures as documentation of clinical outcomes. For example, multiple studies have shown that goniometric measurements of range of motion, an impairment, has poor reliability, and range of motion has little to no correlation with patient disability complaints when examined retrospectively [16–19]. Meanwhile self-report and clinician reports of activity limitations have been found to be reliable and sensitive to change [20,21]. Thus logic suggests that one measures function directly when trying to understand function and measure disability to understand disability. To measure function, disability and QOL outcomes self-report tools are warranted.

Disablement and Choosing/Creating Outcomes Instruments

Construction of general health, condition-specific and region-specific outcomes instruments with foundations in disablement theory should be documented in the literature. Guyatt and colleagues [12] developed a six-stage methodological approach to developing HRQOL instruments: (1) identification of patient population, (2) item generation, (3) item reduction, (4) pretesting, (5) reliability, and (6) validation. All outcomes instruments should have similar methodological origins to be valid instruments. Disablement theory applies in steps 1 and 2 of the process when the patient population is identified and appropriate items are generated for the instrument.

An important criterion when choosing an appropriate instrument is its applicability to a physically active population (step one of Guyatt's methodology). As noted earlier, disablement is a patient-centered process that focuses highly on expectations for function and ability. Therefore, to avoid limitations in an outcomes instrument, the items must assess higher functioning in regards to sport and physical activity. For example, studies have examined the SF-36, a generic HRQOL instrument, and found that it was not as responsive to change as a disease-specific instrument [22–24] and displayed ceiling or floor effects in athletes [25,26]. In general, generic instruments tend to be less responsive than region- or disease-specific instruments, but an examination of the items on the SF-36 demonstrates that the items may be too rudimentary for patients involved in sport, indicating that a generic HRQOL instrument probably should be paired with a disease- or region-specific instrument to assess patient outcomes.

An instrument that purports to measure disablement will have content validity if it measures multiple disablement constructs including QOL. For example, the McGill Pain Questionnaire measures just one construct and therefore only informs the clinician about pain, making it difficult to draw general conclusions about disablement. The Cincinnati Knee Rating System is an example of an instrument that incorporates constructs that measure impairment, function, and disability but excludes items that measure the social aspect of disability and HRQOL. A thorough examination of the content value of an outcomes instrument should be completed by the clinician with the concerns of applicability and patient expectations in mind.

Specific Measurement Properties to Consider When Selecting an Outcome Instrument

Because they commonly are delivered in paper-pencil form, self-reported health outcome instruments are often referred to as surveys. But important health care decisions are based upon these scores, and the consequences have a significant impact in the health care of each patient. Each instrument, therefore, should be treated as a standardized test or examination, similar to board certification or college entrance examinations, where the ability of an examinee is assessed, upon which a decision is made, where a higher score indicates a higher level of ability. But unlike a math test, in health care, the ability being measured is patient function, rather then math ability. The decisions can involve rehabilitation progression, medical referral, cessation of therapy, and ultimately the efficacy of health care interventions. Because of these consequences, these instruments or tests should be held to the same testing standards and undergo the required steps of test construction and reflect appropriate measurement properties before their use in health-related decisions and outcome assessment. These properties commonly are referred to as psychometric properties [27,28], and should be presented in peer-reviewed literature before an instrument's use in clinical practice.

For a clinician, however, sorting through published psychometric research can be a confusing and often a misleading task. Most clinicians are uncertain as to which properties are most important when selecting an instrument. There are some basic guidelines and current recommendations, however, that can allow clinicians to select instruments appropriate for their needs. Assuming that the appropriate preliminary steps have been taken during test construction (eg, identification of the traits or constructs, using a panel of expert judges to establish the content validity, field testing), the instrument can undergo statistical testing of its measurement properties. Two of the most important concepts in supporting the interpretation of a test score are validity and the instrument's measurement capabilities. Furthermore, there are two general approaches to addressing these measurement properties: (1) classical or traditional test analyses and (2) modern measurement theory.

Classical test theory analyses, which have been applied since the early 20th century, are based upon a total test score comprised of the sum of a test's items. Classical test theory typically provides a measure of reliability, validity, item difficulty, and item discrimination (Table 2). Reliability is defined as the amount of error. Reliability is defined as the amount of error expected in any measurement, whether it is systematic or random [28]. It is synonymous with test score consistency or stability. Although important, it often is overemphasized in that if a test demonstrates appropriate test–retest reliability, it often is deemed adequate for use with little additional psychometric analyses.

Validity traditionally has been defined as the degree to which an instrument or test measures what it is designed to measure [29]. Validity further is defined as

Table 2
An overview of measurement properties and validity

Item characteristic	Definition
Difficulty	Derived from the proportion of respondents that answer an item correctly.
Discrimination	The extent to which an item can discriminate between respondents of varying levels of ability.
Validity characteristic	Definition
Construct	The extent to which an instrument measures a theoretical construct, can be convergent or divergent.
Content	Also referred to as "expert" validity, and formerly "face" "validity". Rather than a statistical interpretation, content validity is deemed appropriate by a panel of experts or judges who determine that the items address the appropriate content
Criterion	The correlation of a new test with a criterion measure.
Concurrent criterion	The correlation of a new test with an existing test administered at the same time.
Predictive criterion	The accuracy that test can predict a criterion score obtained at later time.

the degree of confidence placed in the inferences made from the scores of the scales [28] and the soundness of the interpretation [30]. Validity is considered to be one of the most vital properties that should be established [30] and is divided into three broad subcategories to include criterion validity, content validity, and construct validity. Content validity refers to the instrument measuring the trait or construct that it is designed to measure. Each item should represent a component of latent ability trait being assessed. Criterion validity refers to an instrument's correlation with an accepted criterion measure. There are two types of criterion validity: concurrent and predictive. Concurrent refers to the correlation of a new test to that of a criterion test administered at the same time. Predictive criterion validity refers to the capacity to predict a criterion score obtained at a later time. Construct validity, which is the extent to which an instrument measures a theoretic construct, can be distinguished further as convergent (two tests measuring the same trait or construct are correlated highly) or divergent (two tests measuring different traits or constructs are not correlated highly).

Although the listed types of validity are important, the overall approach to test validation has evolved. Previously, if an instrument underwent psychometric testing, and a peer-reviewed publication appeared indicating that an instrument demonstrated appropriate validity, the instrument was often deemed "valid." But the current interpretation of validity is the degree to which accumulated evidence and theory support specific interpretations of test scores entailed by proposed uses of the test [31]. This interpretation of validation represents an ongoing process, requiring multiple pieces of evidence under a unified validity framework [31]. More specifically, the names have been adjusted to criterion evidence, construct evidence, and content evidence to reflect the modern approach to validation. Therefore, one piece of validity evidence does not render a test valid. Rather multiple pieces of evidence, representing various categories of validity evidence, should be compiled when addressing validity.

Responsiveness is synonymous with precision and sensitivity, and it can be defined as the ability of an item to measure a distinct latent trait with minimal error. Responsiveness of an instrument means that it is able to detect small changes within the ability continuum with equal precision.

In addition to establishing validity evidence for an instrument, the measurement capabilities also should be identified. These can include item difficulty, item discrimination, and ceiling and floor effects. The proportion of examinees that answers an item correctly can determine item difficulty. Although in the context of assessing functional ability, the notion of a correct or incorrect response is not an accurate reflection. Consider the following example: 100 people, with varying levels of functional ability, from injured to very healthy, complete a functional rating instrument that uses a Likert scale ranging from 1 through 5 (1 = critical problem, 5 = no problem), and all respond to a certain item with 5 (No problem). The difficulty of that particular item would then be 1 (100 responded no problem ÷ 100 possible responses = 1). In this example, the item would be considered too easy, because everyone responded with the highest possible item score, or in other words, responded correctly, regardless of the ability level. The item therefore would be of little use in measuring level of ability. Item discrimination is the extent that an item can discriminate between examinees with high and low levels of ability. These capabilities can be determined through an item analysis and will allow for the elimination or revision of ineffective items. Ceiling effect occurs when the items on a test cannot assess the high ability range. So as an examinee's ability improves, the test score cannot reflect the change, because items cannot measure high levels of ability precisely. This means that ability ranges only can be measured up to a certain extent. In contrast, a floor effect exists when low ability levels or low health status cannot be measured precisely.

A limitation of classical test theory is that the measures depend on the population sample that is tested. Therefore, the difficulty of an item will change based upon the sample responding. In contrast to traditional testing methods, modern measurement theory, specifically item response theory (IRT), addresses the issues that hinder classical test theory. Item response theory has been used for years in the development of item banks for large testing programs such as college entrance examinations. IRT, however, only recently has been incorporated into health science test construction. IRT treats each item as a test of ability and performs this independent of respondents. Referenced norm standards therefore are eliminated, and different populations can be assessed simultaneously. Furthermore, item responses are calculated independent of other items, so one response does not influence a response on any other item. Items and the ability of the examinees then can be placed on a common metric (high-to-low ability continuum). This allows items to be located to specific ability levels (item difficulty) and identifies the spread of ability between items (item discrimination). It also enables a more accurate assessment of potential ceiling effects of tests. IRT additionally allows for test equating, which determines how scores on different tests correlate with one another. Overall, modern measurement theory provides a better understanding of the capabilities and precision of a test.

Of the properties listed, the issue of instrument precision is of specific interest in sports medicine. Although numerous self-report measures exist for various regions of the body and conditions [32,33], few have been designed and established for use in the physically active population. Most of the instruments contain items that often only address low levels of ability, omitting items that can measure the higher levels of ability demonstrated by physically active clientele. Very active individuals therefore may report very high scores when they have not returned to their preinjury ability level, thus indicating a ceiling effect. Even though they can continue to improve their ability, their scores on an imprecise instrument will not reflect any improvement. With these limitations, there has yet to be a generic self-report measure that has substantial validity evidence to support its use for the physically active.

Overall, when clinicians select an instrument, they should make certain that there is validity evidence to support its use. Furthermore, the instrument should demonstrate the appropriate measurement capabilities such as precision, item difficulty, and item discrimination, along with the identification of floor or ceiling effects for the population being measured. These capabilities can be addressed most accurately through the application of modern measurement theory, which has advantages over traditional analyses. If there is a body of evidence of validity, and the measurement capabilities have been addressed appropriately, then a test instrument has merit for use by a clinician for assessing health outcomes.

SUMMARY

In summary, clear and directed outcomes assessment is an integral part of clinical decision making and moves the state of science forward in sports medicine. Although measurements obtained by clinicians provide valuable data, the scope of disablement requires the incorporation of patient self-report data to fully capture the impact of illness and injury, and responses to treatments on individual patients. Garnering valuable outcomes data requires that clinicians choose instruments that are grounded in disablement theory, designed to measure the ability of a physically active population, and have established psychometric properties. This may mean that there is no ideal instrument for each patient and each setting, specifically the physically active population. The development and evaluation of self-report instruments is an evolving science. The most likely limitation of most current self-report instruments is a ceiling effect, because most instruments were not constructed to measure high functional ability seen in physically active clientele. Most instruments are adequate in measuring lower ability levels, as seen during the initial phases of injury and rehabilitation, and therefore offer valuable information during those phases. A clinician therefore should take into account the constructs that provide the most meaningful information and the context in which the information will be used. This allows for both clinical expertise and patient values to be incorporated into the treatment process, which by definition gets at the heart of what it means to employ evidence-based practice.

References

[1] Sackett D, Straus S, Richardson W, et al. Evidence-based medicine. How to practice and teach EBM. 2nd edition. Edinburgh (Scotland): Churchill Livingstone; 2000.
[2] Pope A, Tarlov A. Disability in America: toward a National agenda for prevention. Washington, DC: National Academy Press; 1991.
[3] Nagi S. Disability concepts revisited: implications for prevention. In: Pope A, Tarlov A, editors. Disability in America: toward a national agenda for prevention. Washington, DC: National Academy Press; 1991. p. 309–27.
[4] Brandt E, Pope A. Enabling America: assessing the role of rehabilitation science and engineering. Washington, DC: National Academy Press; 1997.
[5] World Health Organization. International classification of functioning, disability, and health. Geneva (IL): World Health Organization; 2001.
[6] Verbrugge L, Jette A. The disablement process. Soc Sci Med 1993;38(1):1–14.
[7] Fuhrer M. An agenda for medical rehabilitation outcomes research. Journal of Prosthetics and Orthotics 1995;7(1):35–9.
[8] Whiteneck G. Conceptual models of disability: past, present, and future. In: Field M, Jette A, Martin L, editors. Workshop on disability in America: a new look—summary and background papers. Washington, DC: National Acadamies Press; 2006.
[9] Coffin-Zadai C. Disabling our diagnostic dilemmas. Phys Ther 2007;87(6):641–53.

[10] Wilson R, Cleary P. Linking clinical variables with health-related quality of life: a conceptual model of patient outcomes. JAMA 1995;273(1):59–63.
[11] Ebrahim S. Clinical and public health perspectives and applications of health-related quality-of-life measurements. Soc Sci Med 1995;41(10):1383–94.
[12] Guyatt GH, Feeny DH, Patrick DL. Measuring health-related quality of life. Ann Intern Med 1993;118(8):622–9.
[13] Gill TM, Feinstein AR. A critical appraisal of the quality of quality-of-life measurements. JAMA 1994;272(8):619–26.
[14] McAllister DR, Motamedi AR, Hame SL, et al. Quality-of-life assessment in elite collegiate athletes. Am J Sports Med 2001;29(6):806–10.
[15] Haley S, Coster W, Blinda-Sundberg K. Measuring physical disablement: the contextual challenge. Phys Ther 1994;74(5):443–51.
[16] Barnes CJ, Van Steyn SJ, Fischer RA. The effects of age, sex, and shoulder dominance on range of motion of the shoulder. J Shoulder Elbow Surg 2001;10(3):242–6.
[17] Lowery WD Jr, Horn TJ, Boden SD, et al. Impairment evaluation based on spinal range of motion in normal subjects. J Spinal Disord 1992;5(4):398–402.
[18] Post RB, Leferink VJM. Sagittal range of motion after a spinal fracture: does ROM correlate with functional outcome? Eur Spine J 2004;13(6):489–94.
[19] Roddey TS, Cook KF, O'Malley KJ, et al. The relationship among strength and mobility measures and self-report outcome scores in persons after rotator cuff repair surgery: impairment measures are not enough. J Shoulder Elbow Surg 2005;14(1 Suppl S):95S–8S.
[20] Wilson R, Gansneder B. Measures of functional limitation as predictors of disablement in athletes with acute ankle sprains. J Orthop Sports Phys Ther 2000;30(9):528–35.
[21] Wilson R, Gieck J, Gansneder B, et al. Reliability and responsiveness of disablement measures following acute ankle sprains among athletes. J Orthop Sports Phys Ther 1998;27(5):348–55.
[22] Oga T, Nishimura K, Tsukino M, et al. A comparison of the responsiveness of different generic health status measures in patients with asthma. Qual Life Res 2003;12(5):555–63.
[23] Krahn M, Bremner KE, Tomlinson G, et al. Responsiveness of disease-specific and generic utility instruments in prostate cancer patients. Qual Life Res 2007;16(3):509–22.
[24] Turner JA, Fulton-Kehoe D, Franklin G, et al. Comparison of the Roland-Morris disability questionnaire and generic health status measures: a population-based study of workers' compensation back injury claimants. Spine 2003;28(10):1061–7.
[25] SooHoo NF, Vyas R, Samimi D. Responsiveness of the foot function index, AOFAS clinical rating systems, and SF-36 after foot and ankle surgery. Foot Ankle Int 2006;27(11):930–4.
[26] Campbell H, Rivero-Arias O, Johnston K, et al. Responsiveness of objective, disease-specific, and generic outcome measures in patients with chronic low back pain: an assessment for improving, stable, and deteriorating patients. Spine 2006;31(7):815–22.
[27] Andresen EM. Criteria for assessing the tools of disability outcomes research. Arch Phys Med Rehabil 2000;81(Suppl 2):S15–20.
[28] Streiner DL, Norman GR. Health measurement scales: a practical guide to their development and use. 2nd edition. Oxford (NY): Oxford Medical Publications; 1995.
[29] Vincent WJ. Statistics in kinesiology. 2nd edition. Champaign (IL): Human Kinetics Publishers, Inc; 1999. p. 2.
[30] Thomas JR, Nelson JK. Research methods in physical education. 3rd edition. Champaign (IL): Human Kinetics Publishers, Inc; 1996. p. 214.
[31] American Educational Research Association, American Psychological Association, National Council on Measurement in Education. Standards for educational and psychological testing. Washington, DC: American Educational Research Association; 1999. p. 9–17.
[32] Gonsalves E. Self-report functional -outcome measures in athletic therapy. Athletic Therapy Today 2003;8(6):65–9.
[33] Finch E, Brooks D, Stratford PW, et al. Physical rehabilitation outcome measure: a guide to enhanced clinical decision making. 2nd edition. Hamilton (Ontario): Canadian Physiotherapy Association; 2002.

Clin Sports Med 27 (2008) 353–370

CLINICS IN SPORTS MEDICINE

ELSEVIER
SAUNDERS

Sensorimotor Deficits with Ankle Sprains and Chronic Ankle Instability

Jay Hertel, PhD, ATC

Department of Human Services, University of Virginia, Exercise and Sport Injury Lab,
202 Emmet Street South, Charlottesville, VA 22904-4407, USA

Ankle sprains occur commonly in athletic [1,2], military [3], and occupational [4] settings. Within sports medicine, two recent nationwide injury epidemiology studies found ankle sprains to be the most common injuries suffered by interscholastic [1] and intercollegiate [2] athletes. Ankle sprains are often erroneously considered to be innocuous injuries with no lasting consequences [5], but in fact prolonged symptoms [6,7], self-reported disability [7], diminished physical activity [8], and recurrent injury [9] are commonly reported for months and years after initial injury. Approximately 30% of those suffering an initial lateral ankle sprain develop chronic ankle instability (CAI) or repetitive giving way of the ankle during functional activities [10]. There is also emerging evidence linking severe and repetitive ankle sprains to the development of ankle osteoarthritis [11,12].

Ankle sprains typically involve injury to the lateral ligaments because of hypersupination (a combination of inversion, plantar flexion, and internal rotation) of the not fully loaded rearfoot in relation to the tibia. The most commonly injured ligaments are the anterior talofibular and calcaneofibular ligaments [13]. The initial injury may result in two types of dysfunction, mechanical instability and functional instability, that influence recovery from the acute injury and the development of CAI [14–16]. Mechanical instability is most commonly associated with pathologic joint laxity and has been thoroughly reviewed elsewhere [16]. The focus of this article is on functional instability, which is typically ascribed to sensorimotor, or neuromuscular, deficits that accompany ligamentous injury. The specific aims are to (1) present the traditional theoretic relationships between ankle instability and sensorimotor deficits, (2) concisely review the research evidence demonstrating sensorimotor deficits after acute ankle sprain and with CAI, and (3) refine the theoretic relationships between ankle instability and sensorimotor deficits based on the summary of the research evidence.

E-mail address: jhertel@virginia.edu

0278-5919/08/$ – see front matter
doi:10.1016/j.csm.2008.03.006

TRADITIONAL THEORY OF ANKLE INSTABILITY AND SENSORIMOTOR DEFICITS

Through a series of animal [17] and human [18–21] studies in the 1960s Freeman and colleagues proposed a theory that "functional" (ie, sensorimotor) deficits after joint injuries were attributable to damage to the afferent receptors within the injured ligaments and joint capsule. They specifically referred to this concept as "articular deafferentation" and proposed that when the ankle ligaments were sprained there was disruption not only of the collagenous connective tissue but also to the sensory mechanoreceptors within the ligament. The damage to the sensory receptors was believed to create proprioceptive deficits and prevent the central nervous system's accurate perception of where the ankle joint was in space. This deficit, consequently, would lead to an increased incidence of the ankle giving way into hypersupination because there was inadequate peroneal muscle response to the aberrant ankle positioning. This theory of articular deafferentation went largely unchallenged for more than 25 years.

Freeman's theory of articular deafferentation is still widely cited today when sensorimotor deficits are reported in patients who have ankle sprains or CAI. There are, however, impediments to fully accepting this theory that cannot be ignored. The first is that studies that have aimed to anesthetize the lateral ligaments, and thus directly impair the function of the ligamentous and capsular mechanoreceptors, have failed to consistently show deficits in measures of proprioception [22–24] or postural control [22,24–26]. Interestingly, Konradsen and colleagues [22] used a regional anesthetic block to the entire foot and ankle and found deficits in passive joint position sense, but not active joint position sense, postural control, or peroneal reaction time. They attributed the loss of passive joint position sense to impaired function of the ligamentous mechanoreceptors under anesthesia, although the loss of afferent activity from the plantar cutaneous and intrinsic musculotendinous receptors as other potential causes cannot be summarily dismissed. Konradsen and colleagues [22] attributed the lack of differences in the other measures to be because of the ability to use afferent information from the musculotendinous receptors in the extrinsic ankle muscles that were not affected by their anesthesia technique to "replace" the information lost from the ligamentous receptors. Furthermore, Myers and colleagues [27] reported that deficits in anterior tibialis and peroneal muscle activity during running were equally depressed compared with baseline measures after injection of either an anesthetic or saline into the ankle joint. This finding suggests that any adverse effects may be attributable to edema in the ankle joint rather than actual deafferentation of the lateral ligaments [27]. The lack of substantive changes despite anesthetization of the lateral ankle ligaments is most likely attributable to the tremendous redundancy of sensory information available from articular, musculotendinous, and cutaneous receptors.

The second limitation is that Freeman's theory assumes only a feedback model of articular proprioception and sensorimotor control (Fig. 1). In a feedback-only model, efferent motor control deficits arise only after the damaged

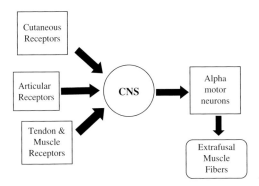

Fig. 1. Feedback-only model of sensorimotor control.

afferents fail to detect that the ankle is in or moving toward a potentially injurious position. The feedback-only model does not take into account the feedforward role of the gamma motoneuron system or the influence of chronic adaptations in the alpha motoneuron pool excitability. Accounting for feedforward mechanisms of motor control is critical because it has been well-documented that there is substantial lower leg muscle activity before initial contact of the foot with the ground during gait and jump landings and, moreover, the peroneal muscles cannot respond quickly enough to prevent a lateral ankle sprain if they operate in a feedback-only manner [28]. The depression of alpha motoneuron pool excitability of the peroneal muscles during resting states among individuals who have CAI [29] also casts considerable doubt on the feedback-only model of articular sensorimotor control.

There is thus a need to re-evaluate the theory of articular deafferentation as it relates to sensorimotor deficits of the ankle after acute sprain and with CAI. By evaluating evidence along a continuum of sensorimotor measures (Fig. 2),

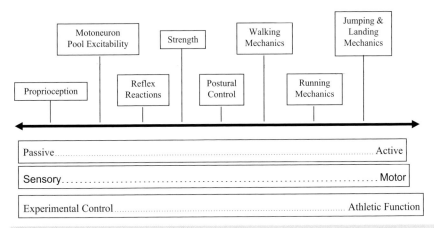

Fig. 2. Spectrum of sensorimotor measures associated with ankle instability.

a more robust theoretic model may be developed to better explain the relationships between these factors and provide a framework for conservative management of ankle instability.

PROPRIOCEPTION

Proprioception allows for the sensation of body movement and position. Although this term is often used (erroneously) in the orthopedic literature to convey the integration of afferent and efferent processes to allow for the dynamic stabilization of joints, proprioception is a purely afferent phenomenon on par with other sensory modalities. Proprioception is most often measured by assessing joint position sense, kinesthesia (sensation of movement), and force sense.

Acute Ankle Sprains

Compared with contralateral uninjured ankles, greater errors in the perception of the position of ankle inversion have been reported in subjects who recently suffered grade II or III ankle sprains [30]. Mean differences of the absolute error in passive joint position sense between injured and uninjured limbs were reported to be 2.5° at 1 week, 1.9° at 3 weeks, and 1.1° at both 6 and 12 weeks' follow-up after acute ankle sprain [30]. No significant differences in passive joint position sense deficits were found at any of the follow-ups between subgroups of subjects who did or did not have documented pathologic laxity, thus suggesting that proprioceptive deficits are present after ankle sprain regardless of the presence of mechanical instability [30]. There do not seem to be any studies that have evaluated kinesthesia or force sense after acute ankle sprain.

Chronic Ankle Instability

Deficits in the threshold to detection of passive motion have been demonstrated in several studies of individuals who have unilateral CAI. Kinesthetic deficits have been shown in the detection of passive plantar flexion [31,32] and inversion [33] within the chronically unstable ankles and contralateral healthy ankles. Refshauge and colleagues [34] demonstrated deficits in detecting inversion and eversion, but not plantar flexion and dorsiflexion movement [35], between CAI and control groups. More recently, De Noronha and colleagues [36] reported no differences in assessment of passive movement into inversion or eversion within ankles of subjects with unilateral CAI, or between CAI and control groups.

Konradsen and Magnusson [37] demonstrated deficits in recreating inversion positioning (active position sense) among individuals who had unilateral mechanical instability compared with their contralateral uninvolved ankle (0.5°) and compared with healthy control subjects (0.8°), whereas Nakasa and colleagues [38] found individuals who had unilateral CAI to have side-to-side differences of 1.0° and controls had side-to-side differences of 0.2° for inversion replication. Studies identifying no differences between CAI and control groups in active position sense have also been reported [39–41]. Deficits in passive joint position sense in inversion have also been reported between CAI and control groups with deficits ranging from 0.3° to 0.4° [42].

Assuming that statistically significant deficits in joint position sense exist, the clinical importance of the magnitude of these mean differences ($\leq 2.5°$ after acute sprain, $\leq 1°$ with CAI) must be addressed. Konradsen and Voigt [43] applied these magnitudes of joint position errors attributable to CAI to a gait simulation study and postulated that such deficits would lead an individual who had a proprioceptive deficit attributable to CAI to be much more likely to suffer an ankle sprain mechanism because of improper foot positioning at initial contact compared with healthy individuals.

Another area of proprioception that has received attention in the ankle instability literature in recent years has been force sense. Force sense represents the ability of an individual to recreate specific force outputs in particular muscle groups. Poor force sense is believed to be caused by proprioceptive deficits stemming from dysfunction of the muscle spindles and Golgi tendon organs in the musculotendinous units crossing an injured joint. Diminished eversion force sense has been reported between involved and uninvolved ankles in subjects who had unilateral CAI [44]. Additionally, a significant correlation between eversion force sense and CAI status has been identified [41].

Together the deficits identified in kinesthesia, joint position sense, and force sense indicate that it is likely that there are afferent proprioceptive deficits associated with ankle instability. It must be emphasized, however, that these measures are not strictly afferent assessments because they all rely on conscious supraspinal perception of peripheral somatosensory information. It is thus not possible to conclusively determine if deficits in these measures related to ankle instability represent peripheral afferent dysfunction, central nervous system alterations at the spinal or supraspinal levels, or both.

MOTONEURON POOL EXCITABILITY

Arthrogenic muscle inhibition has been defined as a continuing reflex reaction of the musculature surrounding a joint after distension or damage to the structures of that joint [45]. Arthrogenic muscle inhibition is measured by assessing motoneuron pool excitability of a specific muscle group. This assessment is not a direct measure of muscle contraction output, but rather an estimation of how much of the alpha motoneuron pool for a specific muscle group is available and, in some measures, activated.

Acute Ankle Sprains

There do not seem to be any studies that have examined motoneuron pool excitability after acute ankle sprains using the robust assessment methods used in the CAI studies described below.

Chronic Ankle Instability

Diminished H-reflex/M-response ratios have been demonstrated in the peroneus longus and soleus muscles of individuals who have CAI [29]. Interestingly, using measures of the central activation ration, inhibition of the quadriceps, and facilitation (increased alpha motoneuron pool excitability) of the antagonist hamstring muscles have also been reported among those who have CAI [46]. Together, these findings provide evidence of altered motoneuron pool excitability related to CAI status not only in muscles that cross the ankle joint but also in proximal leg muscles. These differences indicate spinal level motor control deficits associated with CAI.

REFLEX REACTIONS TO INVERSION PERTURBATION

Several researchers have assessed muscular response to unexpected ankle inversion perturbations in an attempt to assess sensorimotor deficits associated with ankle instability. Considerable methodological differences exist across these studies, but in general a research subject stands on a trapdoor platform that is triggered to unexpectedly drop one of the subject's ankles into inversion (and sometimes plantar flexion or internal rotation too). Surface electromyography is used to assess the time from trapdoor initiation to reflexive muscle response.

Acute Ankle Sprains

In a study comparing recently sprained and contralateral uninjured ankles, no differences in peroneal muscle reaction time to sudden inversion were identified at 3, 6, or 12 weeks postinjury [30]. No studies investigating differences in muscle reaction time between groups with and without recent ankle sprains were identified.

Chronic Ankle Instability

There are conflicting results in the literature pertaining to muscle reaction time to inversion perturbation related to CAI. Several studies [47–52] have identified delayed reaction time of the peroneal muscles in limbs with a chronically unstable ankle, although several other studies [53–58] have not identified such differences. This discrepancy may be because of methodological differences across studies relating to varying inclusion criteria of subjects who have CAI; differences in the rate, direction, and angle of ankle perturbation allowed by the trapdoor mechanisms; and use of different EMG processing techniques to determine the onset of reflexive muscle activation.

If we assume that delayed peroneal reflex responses are in fact present among individuals who have CAI, these may be attributable to local proprioceptive deficits or spinal level alterations in motor control.

MUSCLE STRENGTH

It is often assumed that lateral ankle instability is associated with peroneal muscle weakness; however, there is not overwhelming experimental evidence to support this notion [59]. In addition to the peroneals, studies have also investigated the strength of the other prime movers about the ankle. If muscle strength deficits do exist after ankle sprain, the physiologic mechanism of such deficits is not readily apparent. Although mechanical damage to the peroneal tendons does occasionally occur with lateral ankle sprains [60], muscle or tendon strains are certainly not common. A more plausible explanation for muscle dysfunction may be the changes in alpha motoneuron pool excitability because of arthrogenic muscle inhibition discussed earlier.

Acute Ankle Sprains

A significant deficit in isometric strength for ankle eversion has been reported in acutely sprained ankles in comparison to contralateral uninjured ankles 3 weeks after injury; however, no deficits were identified at 6- and 12-week follow-up [30]. Similarly, Holme and colleagues [61] reported significant side-to-side deficits in isometric strength for ankle eversion, inversion, plantar flexion, and dorsiflexion at 6 weeks post–ankle sprain, but differences were no longer present at 4-month follow-up. The resolution of these strength deficits occurred regardless of the performance of supervised rehabilitation [61]. Alterations in the activation of the gluteal muscles has also been reported after severe ankle sprain, indicating that proximal muscles may also be affected after ankle injury [62,63].

Chronic Ankle Instability

There is conflicting evidence regarding the presence of eversion strength deficits with CAI. Several studies [64–66] have identified eversion strength deficits, but others [33,67–69] have not. Inversion strength deficits with CAI have also been reported by some authors [66,70,71] The mechanism of inversion strength deficits has been suggested to be a reflexive inhibition of the muscles that can concentrically contract to produce the motion that caused the initial joint injury [71]. Two recent studies [72,73] have identified deficits in plantar flexion strength in association with CAI. These deficits may be related to the inhibition of the soleus muscle with CAI described earlier [29].

Strength deficits have also been identified in the performance of hip extension and hip abduction in individuals who have CAI [72,74,75]. The mechanism of such deficits is not clear, although it would seem to be neurally mediated. Altered activation of the gluteus maximus muscle has been identified after severe ankle sprain [62,63]. It is possible that hip muscle function is altered after ankle sprain as a protective mechanism for the injured limb. Failure to restore normal hip muscle function may, however, have lasting consequences. In an intriguing finding, Kramer and colleagues [76] recently reported that individuals who suffered anterior cruciate ligament (ACL) injuries were more likely than healthy controls to have a history of previous ankle sprain ipsilaterally to the injured knee. There is mounting evidence relating motor control of the hip to ACL injury risk [77] so the presence of lasting hip muscle dysfunction after ankle sprain may be an important deficit for clinicians to target during rehabilitation.

Any strength deficits associated with CAI are likely attributable to differences in motoneuron pool excitability and recruitment rather than actual musculotendinous unit damage. Such deficits would seem to indicate spinal, or possibly supraspinal, motor control deficits.

POSTURAL CONTROL

Measures of balance, or postural control, during single limb stance have frequently been used to estimate sensorimotor function in individuals who have lateral ankle instability. Postural control requires the integration of somatosensory, visual, and vestibular afferent information and appropriate efferent responses to control muscles in the trunk and extremities in an effort to maintain balance. Researchers have used noninstrumented and instrumented assessments of postural control in relation to ankle instability. Two systematic reviews [78,79] have recently been published that exhaustively cover this topic; a more concise version is presented here.

Acute Ankle Sprains

Postural control deficits have been conclusively shown to be present in individuals after acute ankle sprain [78]. There seem to be postural control deficits on the involved and uninvolved limbs for up to 1 week after acute ankle sprain [80]. These deficits indicate an unambiguous change in centrally mediated sensorimotor control after an acute ankle injury. The deficits on the involved limbs remain for a longer period of time than the uninvolved limbs [80], but similar to strength deficits, any side-to-side differences seem to resolve within a few months after injury [61,81]. Deficits in dynamic postural control have also been demonstrated after acute ankle sprain using the Star Excursion Balance Test [82].

Chronic Ankle Instability

There are conflicting results in the literature regarding static postural control deficits associated with CAI [78], especially with traditional center-of-pressure–based measures of static postural control derived from instrumented force plates [78]. More sophisticated measures of postural control estimating the time-to-boundary of support during single limb stance have recently identified deficits more clearly [83,84]. This method of assessment seems to indicate that individuals who have unilateral CAI have measurable deficits when standing on both their involved and uninvolved limbs in comparison to healthy controls [83].

Several studies [85–89] have also been performed to assess the ability of subjects to maintain their postural control after landing from a jump using time-to-stabilization measures. In this experimental setup, subjects are asked to "stick" their single limb landing from a jump onto a force plate and then maintain their balance. The dependent measure involves the time it takes to reach and maintain a stable posture after landing. Deficits have been consistently shown in subjects who have CAI compared with control [85–89].

Various noninstrumented measures of static balance have also been used to identify postural control deficits associated with CAI [19,20,32,90]. The most basic of these simply involves either patient or clinician judgment of whether it is more difficult to maintain balance on the involved or uninvolved limb [19,20,32]. A more robust measure is the Balance Error Scoring System (BESS), which uses a simple scoring system by counting balance errors during various stance conditions [91]. The BESS was originally developed to assess for balance deficits associated with cerebral concussion [91], but has also been shown to be able to detect deficits related to CAI [90].

A noninstrumented assessment of dynamic postural control, the Star Excursion Balance Test, has been used to identify sensorimotor deficits associated with CAI [92–94]. This test requires a subject to maintain balance on one leg while reaching as far as possible in one of eight prescribed directions with the opposite limb. On maximal reach, the subject must lightly tap the toe of the reach limb on the ground and then return to a bilateral stance position. The reach distance (normalized to subject leg length) is then measured and serves as a measure of performance. In addition to identifying deficits related to CAI, performance on this test has also been shown to improve following rehabilitation for CAI [95]. Compared with the bilateral deficits identified with instrumented testing of static postural control, only deficits on the involved limb have been identified with the Star Excursion Balance Test. In lieu of testing all eight reach directions, it is now recommend that only three reach directions (anterior, posteromedial, posterolateral) be tested because of the redundant information provided by the different directions (Fig. 3) [94].

The bilateral deficits in static postural control found after acute ankle sprain and with unilateral CAI indicate spinal or supraspinal mechanisms of motor control deficits. Further evidence of the central mediation of postural control is evidenced by the finding of a crossover effect with rehabilitation. Individuals who had unilateral CAI who only performed rehabilitation exercises on their involved limb were found to have bilateral improvements in postural control [95].

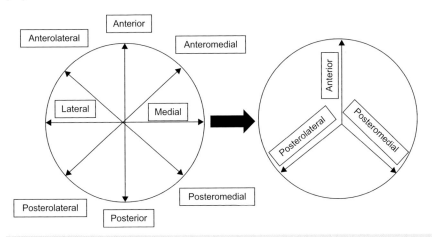

Fig. 3. Reach directions for left limb stance of the Star Excursion Balance Test. Directions are labeled based on the reach direction from the stance limb. On the left, the original eight reach directions of the star. On the right, the currently recommended three reach directions (peace sign).

GAIT

There have been relatively few studies published that have examined gait deficits associated with acute ankle sprain or CAI.

Acute Ankle Sprains

Parameters of walking gait, such as stride speed, have been found to be altered in the days and weeks after acute lateral ankle sprain [96,97]. Because limping is obvious to the naked eye after an individual has suffered an acute ankle sprain, it should not be surprising that there are limited instrumented data in this population.

Chronic Ankle Instability

Spaulding and colleagues [98] reported that individuals who had chronically unstable ankles were more plantar flexed at initial contact than controls. Subjects who have CAI have also been reported to have increased plantar pressures on the lateral aspect of their feet during walking [99]. Likewise, a significant delay to the time to peak force under the central and lateral forefoot and an increase in the relative forces under the midfoot and lateral forefoot in subjects who have CAI compared with controls has been reported during walking [100].

Monaghan and colleagues [101] demonstrated that individuals who had CAI were significantly more inverted in the frontal plane compared with controls before and after initial contact. Additionally, the joint angular velocity was significantly higher at heel strike in the CAI group compared with a control group [101]. Additionally, during the early stance phase of gait, CAI subjects seemed to use an evertor muscle moment working concentrically compared with an invertor muscle moment working eccentrically in controls [101]. In a follow-up study by Delahunt and colleagues [102], the inversion kinematic differences associated with CAI were confirmed and CAI subjects were also found to have increased peroneus longus EMG activity immediately after heel strike in comparison to controls. The authors attributed these findings to a change in feedforward motor control associated with CAI [101,102].

JUMP LANDINGS

High-level sensorimotor function in individuals who have CAI has been assessed with various kinesiologic measures during jump landings. Assessment during such activities is advocated by researchers because landing from a jump is a frequent mechanism of lateral ankle sprain.

Acute Ankle Sprains

Not surprisingly, there do not seem to be any studies that have examined jump landing performance in subjects recovering from acute ankle sprains.

Chronic Ankle Instability

Subjects who have CAI have been shown to have different kinetic and kinematic patterns during jump landings compared with controls [103,104]. CAI subjects used more knee flexion range of motion during landing than controls

[103] and reached peak ground reaction forces more quickly after landing than controls [104]. Subjects who had CAI also demonstrated significantly less peroneal EMG activity and were in a more inverted position before initial contact [105]. On landing, CAI subjects reached their peak vertical ground reaction force faster than controls [105]. Additionally, individuals who had CAI who exhibited greater angles of ankle inversion during a drop landing were found to use greater cocontraction of the ankle dorsiflexor and plantar flexor muscles, which in turn was associated with greater impact force at initial contact compared with controls [106].

The differences in movement characteristics before landing indicate feedforward control differences, governed by either spinal or supraspinal mechanisms, associated with CAI.

CONTEMPORARY THEORY: ANKLE INSTABILITY AND SENSORIMOTOR DEFICITS

Building from Freeman's original theory of joint deafferentation after ankle ligament injury that is based on a feedback-only model of proprioceptive and efferent motor control deficits, we are able to contextualize the current body of literature to form a more comprehensive theoretic model that encompasses both feedback and feedforward mechanisms of motor control deficits related to ankle instability (Fig. 4). Direct evidence to show mechanoreceptor deficits after ankle ligament injury remains absent; however, by examining the spectrum of sensorimotor deficits identified with ankle instability a clearer understanding of the scope of the pathophysiology emerges. The initial ligamentous injury clearly results in immediate deficits in ankle proprioception (as assessed with current methodology), integrated sensorimotor function, and efferent muscle activity. The presence of bilateral postural control deficits after acute ankle sprain and with CAI provides obvious evidence of central changes in sensorimotor control. This information coupled with evidence of altered alpha motoneuron pool excitability in individuals who have CAI indicates that

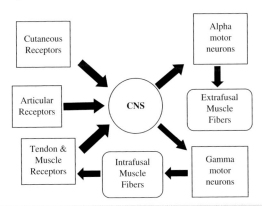

Fig. 4. Model of sensorimotor control encompassing feedback and feedforward mechanisms.

spinal-level motor control mechanisms are clearly altered. Because propriocep-tive measures in vivo require conscious perception of peripheral joint and mus-cle information, it is reasonable to assume that in some way supraspinal aspects of motor control are also altered with ankle instability.

Attempting to pinpoint the initial physiologic site of pathology resulting in this spectrum of sensorimotor dysfunction may be futile. It is apparent that al-though initial sensorimotor deficits may be attributable to the loss of structural ligamentous integrity, edema, or pain immediately after ankle sprain, some as-pects of sensorimotor dysfunction remain after ligament healing and resolution of edema and pain in individuals who go on to develop CAI. A more important effort in clinical management of ankle sprains and CAI is identifying potential points of intervention to alleviate the sensorimotor deficits. The spectrum of sensorimotor deficits (see Fig. 2) may be used as a map to identify potential sites of conservative intervention.

The concept of performing proprioceptive exercises has been thoroughly de-bunked by Ashton-Miller and colleagues [107] in their eloquent article empha-sizing the strictly afferent nature of proprioception so this is unlikely to be a successful site for physiologic intervention. The use of isolated ankle strength training seems to have some beneficial effects on a range of sensorimotor func-tion [108], but the mechanism of action of such training may not be fully suc-cessful if strength deficits are attributable to arthrogenic muscle inhibition caused by spinal level adaptations. Use of interventions, such as cryotherapy and transcutaneous electrical nerve stimulation, has been shown to have disin-hibitory effects in experimental studies using artificial joint effusion [109]. The potential use of these modalities for disinhibitory purposes in patients who have ankle instability has not yet been studied, but holds potential.

Postural control training after acute ankle sprains has clearly been shown to have advantageous effects in the prevention of recurrent ankle sprains [61,110–112]. Likewise, such training in individuals who have CAI has resulted in im-proved sensorimotor and self-reported function [95,113,114]. The physiologic mechanism of this training stimulus, however, has not been clearly identified. It is possible that postural control training is able to create adaptations in the spinal and supraspinal levels of motor control [115]. It is conceivable that pos-tural control training allows the central nervous system to retune the way it in-terprets somatosensory information. There are clearly redundant degrees of freedom in the sensorimotor system so even the complete loss of afferent infor-mation from an injured ligament may be accommodated for with afferent information from receptors in surrounding ligaments, joint capsule, musculo-tendinous units, and skin.

One intriguing development in the ankle instability literature is the use of stochastic resonance as an adjunct to postural control training. Ross [116,117] have reported improved outcomes in patients who had CAI who per-formed postural control training with stochastic resonance stimulation com-pared with those who trained without this adjunct. They surmise that stochastic resonance may be beneficial because it floods the central nervous system with extraneous somatosensory noise and forces the central nervous system to develop adaptive strategies to more clearly detect relevant afferent information from peripheral mechanoreceptors. This theory seems to indicate that improvement is related to the enhanced tuning of the central nervous system to afferent signals.

Last, the contemporary theory linking sensorimotor deficits to ankle instability must encompass the feedforward alterations identified in the studies of gait and landing and in those that have identified motor control deficits in joints proximal to the ankle. The presence of kinematic and electromyographic changes before initial contact during gait and landing indicates that adaptations in motor patterns have occurred regardless of whether or not the ankle is approaching a potentially injurious situation. The feedforward loop mediated by the gamma motoneuron system between the central nervous system and the muscle spindles is the likely physiologic mechanism by which these alterations are governed [118]. An enhanced understanding of the effects of ankle ligament injury on gamma motoneuron function and subsequent interaction with the alpha motoneuron system is needed to better target interventions aimed at resolution of feedforward changes in motor control related to ankle instability.

SUMMARY

Alterations in a spectrum of sensorimotor deficits have been identified in individuals after acute ankle sprain and with chronic ankle instability. It is apparent that conscious perception of afferent somatosensory information, reflex responses, and efferent motor control deficits are present with ankle instability. The specific origin of these deficits local to the ankle ligaments or at the spinal or supraspinal levels of motor control have yet to be fully elucidated; however, it is clear that both feedback and feedforward mechanisms of motor control are altered with ankle instability. Clinicians may use this information when identifying specific interventions aimed at restoring sensorimotor function in patients who have ankle instability.

References

[1] Fernandez WG, Yard EE, Comstock RD. Epidemiology of lower extremity injuries among U.S. high school athletes. Acad Emerg Med 2007;14(7):641–5.

[2] Hootman JM, Dick R, Agel J. Epidemiology of collegiate injuries for 15 sports: summary and recommendations for injury prevention initiatives. J Athl Train 2007;42(2):311–9.

[3] Almeida SA, Williams KM, Shaffer RA, et al. Epidemiological patterns of musculoskeletal injuries and physical training. Med Sci Sports Exerc 1999;31(8):1176–82.

[4] Praemer A, Furner S, Rice DP. Musculoskeletal conditions in the United States. Rosemont (IL): American Academy of Orthopaedic Surgeons; 1999.

[5] McKay GD, Goldie PA, Payne WR, et al. Ankle injuries in basketball: injury rate and risk factors. Br J Sports Med 2001;35:103–8.

[6] Braun BL. Effects of ankle sprain in a general clinic population 6 to 18 months after medical evaluation. Arch Fam Med 1999;8:143–8.

[7] Anandacoomarasamy A, Barnsley L. Long term outcomes of inversion ankle injuries. Br J Sports Med 2005;39(3):e14.

[8] Verhagen RA, de Keizer G, van Dijk CN. Long-term follow-up of inversion trauma of the ankle. Arch Orthop Trauma Surg 1995;114:92–6.

[9] Yeung MS, Chan KM, So CH, et al. An epidemiological survey on ankle sprain. Br J Sports Med 1994;28:112–6.

[10] Itay SA, Ganel H, Horoszowski H, et al. Clinical and functional status following lateral ankle sprains. Orthop Rev 1982;11:73–6.

[11] Gross P, Marti B. Risk of degenerative ankle joint disease in volleyball players: study of former elite athletes. Int J Sports Med 1999;20:58–63.

[12] Valderrabano V, Hintermann B, Horisberger M, et al. Ligamentous posttraumatic ankle osteoarthritis. Am J Sports Med 2006;34:612–20.

[13] Fallat L, Grimm DJ, Saracco JA. Sprained ankle syndrome: prevalence and analysis of 639 acute injuries. J Foot Ankle Surg 1998;37(4):280–5.

[14] Hertel J. Functional instability following lateral ankle sprain. Sports Med 2000;29: 361–71.

[15] Hertel J. Functional anatomy, pathomechanics, and pathophysiology of lateral ankle instability. J Athl Train 2002;37:364–75.

[16] Hubbard TJ, Hertel J. Mechanical contributions to chronic lateral ankle instability. Sports Med 2006;36:263–77.

[17] Freeman MA, Wyke B. The innervation of the ankle joint. An anatomical and histological study in the cat. Acta Anat 1967;68(3):321–33.

[18] Freeman MA. Treatment of ruptures of the lateral ligament of the ankle. J Bone Joint Surg Br 1965;47(4):661–8.

[19] Freeman MA. Instability of the foot after injuries to the lateral ligament of the ankle. J Bone Joint Surg Br 1965;47(4):669–77.

[20] Freeman MA, Dean MR, Hanham IW. The etiology and prevention of functional instability of the foot. J Bone Joint Surg Br 1965;47(4):678–85.

[21] Freeman MA, Wyke B. Articular reflexes at the ankle joint: an electromyographic study of normal and abnormal influences of ankle-joint mechanoreceptors upon reflex activity in the leg muscles. Br J Surg 1967;54(12):990–1001.

[22] Konradsen L, Ravn JB, Sørensen AI. Proprioception at the ankle: the effect of anaesthetic blockade of ligament receptors. J Bone Joint Surg Br 1993;75(3):433–6.

[23] Hertel J, Guskiewicz KM, Kahler DM, et al. Effect of lateral ankle joint anesthesia on center of balance, postural sway, and joint position sense. J Sport Rehabil 1996;5:111–9.

[24] Feuerbach JW, Grabiner MD, Koh TJ, et al. Effect of an ankle orthosis and ankle ligament anesthesia on ankle joint proprioception. Am J Sports Med 1994;22:223–9.

[25] DeCarlo MS, Talbot RW. Evaluation of ankle proprioception following injection of the anterior talofibular ligament. J Orthop Sports Phys Ther 1986;8:70–6.

[26] Riemann BL, Myers JB, Stone DA, et al. Effect of lateral ankle ligament anesthesia on single-leg stance stability. Med Sci Sports Exerc 2004;36(3):388–96.

[27] Myers JB, Riemann BL, Hwang JH, et al. Effect of peripheral afferent alteration of the lateral ankle ligaments on dynamic stability. Am J Sports Med 2003;31(4):498–506.

[28] Konradsen L, Voigt M, Højsgaard C. Ankle inversion injuries. The role of the dynamic defense mechanism. Am J Sports Med 1997;25(1):54–8.

[29] McVey ED, Palmieri RM, Docherty CL, et al. Arthrogenic muscle inhibition in the leg muscles of subjects exhibiting functional ankle instability. Foot Ankle Int 2005;26:1055–61.

[30] Konradsen L, Olesen S, Hansen HM. Ankle sensorimotor control and eversion strength after acute ankle inversion injuries. Am J Sports Med 1998;26(1):72–7.

[31] Garn SN, Newton RA. Kinesthetic awareness in subjects with multiple ankle sprains. Phys Ther 1988;68:1667–71.

[32] Forkin DM, Koczur C, Battle R, et al. Evaluation of kinesthetic deficits indicative of balance control in gymnasts with unilateral chronic ankle sprains. J Orthop Sports Phys Ther 1996;23:245–50.

[33] Lentell G, Baas B, Lopez D, et al. The contributions of proprioceptive deficits, muscle function, and anatomic laxity to functional instability of the ankle. J Orthop Sports Phys Ther 1995;21:206–15.

[34] Refshauge KM, Kilbreath SL, Raymond J. Deficits in detection of inversion and eversion movements among subjects with recurrent ankle sprains. J Orthop Sports Phys Ther 2003;33(4):166–73.

[35] Refshauge KM, Kilbreath SL, Raymond J. The effect of recurrent ankle inversion sprain and taping on proprioception at the ankle. Med Sci Sports Exerc 2000;32(1):10–5.

[36] de Noronha M, Refshauge KM, Kilbreath SL, et al. Loss of proprioception or motor control is not related to functional ankle instability: an observational study. Aust J Physiother 2007;53(3):193–8.

[37] Konradsen L, Magnusson P. Increased inversion angle replication error in functional ankle instability. Knee Surg Sports Traumatol Arthrosc 2000;8(4):246–51.

[38] Nakasa T, Fukuhara K, Adachi N, et al. The deficit of joint position sense in the chronic unstable ankle as measured by inversion angle replication error. Arch Orthop Trauma Surg 2008;128(5):445–9.

[39] Gross MT. Effects of recurrent lateral ankle sprains on active and passive judgments of joint position. Phys Ther 1987;67:1505–9.

[40] Brown C, Ross S, Mynark R, et al. Assessing functional ankle instability with joint position sense, time to stabilization, and electromyography. J Sport Rehabil 2004;13: 122–34.

[41] Docherty CL, Arnold BL, Hurwitz S. Contralateral force sense deficits are related to the presence of functional ankle instability. J Orthop Res 2006;24(7):1412–9.

[42] Fu AS, Hui-Chan CW. Ankle joint proprioception and postural control in basketball players with bilateral ankle sprains. Am J Sports Med 2005;33(8):1174–82.

[43] Konradsen L, Voigt M. Inversion injury biomechanics in functional ankle instability: a cadaver study of simulated gait. Scand J Med Sci Sports 2002;12(6):329–36.

[44] Arnold BL, Docherty CL. Low-load eversion force sense, self-reported ankle instability, and frequency of giving way. J Athl Train 2006;41(3):233–8.

[45] Hopkins JT, Ingersoll CD. Arthrogenic muscle inhibition: a limiting factor in joint rehabilitation. J Sport Rehabil 2000;9:135–59.

[46] Sedory EJ, McVey ED, Cross KM, et al. Arthrogenic muscle response of the quadriceps and hamstrings with chronic ankle instability. J Athl Train 2007;42(3):355–60.

[47] Karlsson J, Andréasson GO. The effect of external ankle support in chronic lateral ankle joint instability: an electromyographic study. Am J Sports Med 1992;20:257–61.

[48] Brunt D, Anderson JC, Huntsman B, et al. Postural responses to lateral perturbation in healthy subjects and ankle sprain patients. Med Sci Sports Exerc 1992;24:171–6.

[49] Konradsen L, Ravn JB. Ankle instability caused by prolonged peroneal reaction time. Acta Orthop Scand 1990;61:388–90.

[50] Lynch SA, Eklund U, Gottlieb D, et al. Electromyographic latency changes in the ankle musculature during inversion moments. Am J Sports Med 1996;24:362–9.

[51] Lofvenberg R, Karrholm J, Sundelin G, et al. Prolonged reaction time in patients with chronic lateral instability of the ankle. Am J Sports Med 1995;23:414–7.

[52] Vaes P, Van Gheluwe B, Duquet W. Control of acceleration during sudden ankle supination in people with unstable ankles. J Orthop Sports Phys Ther 2001;31(12):741–52.

[53] Isakov E, Mizrahi J, Solzi P, et al. Response of the peroneal muscles to sudden inversion stress during standing. Int J Sport Biomech 1986;2:100–6.

[54] Nawoczenski DA, Cook TM, Saltzman CL. The effect of foot orthotics on three-dimensional kinematics of the leg and rearfoot during running. J Orthop Sports Phys Ther 1995;21: 317–27.

[55] Johnson MB, Johnson CL. Electromyographic response of peroneal muscles in surgical and nonsurgical injured ankles during sudden inversion. J Orthop Sports Phys Ther 1993;18: 497–501.

[56] Ebig M, Lephart SM, Burdett RG, et al. The effect of sudden inversion stress on EMG activity of the peroneal and tibialis anterior muscles in the chronically unstable ankle. J Orthop Sports Phys Ther 1997;26:73–7.

[57] Fernandes N, Allison GT, Hopper D. Peroneal latency in normal and injured ankles at varying angles of perturbation. Clin Orthop 2000;375:193–201.

[58] Vaes P, Duquet W, Van Gheluwe B. Peroneal reaction times and eversion motor response in healthy and unstable ankles. J Athl Train 2002;37(4):475–80.

[59] Kaminski TW, Hartsell HD. Factors contributing to chronic ankle instability: a strength perspective. J Athl Train 2002;37(4):394–405.

[60] Karlsson J, Wiger P. Longitudinal split of the peroneus brevis tendon and lateral ankle instability: treatment of concomitant lesions. J Athl Train. 2002;37(4):463–6.

[61] Holme E, Magnusson SP, Becher K, et al. The effect of supervised rehabilitation on strength, postural sway, position sense and re-injury risk after acute ankle ligament sprain. Scand J Med Sci Sports 1999;9:104–9.

[62] Bullock-Saxton JE. Sensory changes associated with severe ankle sprain. Scand J Rehabil Med 1995;27(3):161–7.

[63] Bullock-Saxton JE, Janda V, Bullock MI. The influence of ankle sprain injury on muscle activation during hip extension. Int J Sports Med 1994;15(6):330–4.

[64] Tropp H. Pronator weakness in functional instability of the ankle joint. Int J Sports Med 1986;7:291–4.

[65] Bush KW. Predicting ankle sprain. J Man Manip Ther 1996;4:54–8.

[66] Hartsell HD, Spaulding SJ. Eccentric/concentric ratios at selected velocities for the invertor and evertor muscles of the chronically unstable ankle. Br J Sports Med 1999;33:255–8.

[67] Lentell GL, Katzmann LL, Walters MR. The relationship between muscle function and ankle instability. J Orthop Sports Phys Ther 1990;11:605–11.

[68] Bernier JN, Perrin DH, Rijke A. Effect of unilateral functional instability of the ankle on postural sway and inversion and eversion strength. J Athl Train 1997;32:226–32.

[69] Kaminski TW, Perrin DH, Gansneder BM. Eversion strength analysis of uninjured and functionally unstable ankles. J Athl Train 1999;34:239–45.

[70] Ryan L. Mechanical stability, muscle strength, and proprioception in the functionally unstable ankle. Aust J Physiother 1994;40:41–7.

[71] Wilkerson GB, Pinerola JJ, Caturano RW. Invertor vs. evertor peak torque and power deficiencies associated with lateral ankle ligament injury. J Orthop Sports Phys Ther 1997;26(2):78–86.

[72] Hubbard TJ, Kramer LC, Denegar CR, et al. Contributing factors to chronic ankle instability. Foot Ankle Int 2007;28(3):343–54.

[73] Fox J, Docherty CL, Schrader J, et al. Eccentric plantar-flexor torque deficits in participants with functional ankle instability. J Athl Train 2008;43(1):51–4.

[74] Nicholas JA, Strizak AM, Veras G. A study of thigh muscle weakness in different pathological states of the lower extremity. Am J Sports Med 1976;4:241–8, 74.

[75] Friel K, McLean N, Myers C, et al. Ipsilateral hip abductor weakness after inversion ankle sprain. J Athl Train 2006;41(1):74–8.

[76] Kramer LC, Denegar CR, Buckley WE, et al. Factors associated with anterior cruciate ligament injury history in female athletes. J Sports Med Phys Fitness 2007;47(4):446–54.

[77] Hewett TE, Myer GD, Ford KR. Anterior cruciate ligament injuries in female athletes: part 1, mechanisms and risk factors. Am J Sports Med 2006;34(2):299–311.

[78] McKeon PO, Hertel J. Systematic review of postural control and lateral ankle instability, part 1: can deficits be detected with instrumented testing? J Athl Train 2008;43(3):293–304.

[79] McKeon PO, Hertel J. Systematic review of postural control and lateral ankle instability, part 2: is balance training clinically effective? J Athl Train 2008;43(3):305–15.

[80] Evans T, Hertel J, Sebastianelli W. Bilateral deficits in postural control following lateral ankle sprain. Foot Ankle Int 2004;25(11):833–9.

[81] Hertel J, Buckley WE, Denegar CR. Serial testing of postural control after acute lateral ankle sprain. J Athl Train 2001;36(4):363–8.

[82] Akbari M, Karimi H, Farahini H, et al. Balance problems after unilateral lateral ankle sprains. J Rehabil Res Dev 2006;43(7):819–24.

[83] Hertel J, Olmsted-Kramer LC. Deficits in time-to-boundary measures of postural control with chronic ankle instability. Gait Posture 2007;25:33–9.

[84] McKeon PO, Hertel J. Spatiotemporal postural control deficits are present in those with chronic ankle instability. BMC Musculoskelet Disord, in press.

[85] Ross SE, Guskiewicz KM. Examination of static and dynamic postural stability in individuals with functionally stable and unstable ankles. Clin J Sport Med 2004;14(6):332–8.

[86] Ross SE, Guskiewicz KM, Yu B. Single-leg jump-landing stabilization times in subjects with functionally unstable ankles. J Athl Train 2005;40(4):298–304.

[87] Wikstrom EA, Tillman MD, Borsa PA. Detection of dynamic stability deficits in subjects with functional ankle instability. Med Sci Sports Exerc 2005;37(2):169–75.

[88] Wikstrom EA, Tillman MD, Chmielewski TL, et al. Dynamic postural stability deficits in subjects with self-reported ankle instability. Med Sci Sports Exerc 2007;39(3):397–402.

[89] Ross SE, Guskiewicz KM, Gross MT, et al. Assessment tools for identifying functional limitations associated with functional ankle instability. J Athl Train 2008;43(1):44–50.

[90] Docherty CL, Valovich McLeod TC, Shultz SJ. Postural control deficits in participants with functional ankle instability as measured by the balance error scoring system. Clin J Sport Med 2006;16(3):203–8.

[91] Riemann BL, Guskiewicz KM. Effects of mild head injury on postural stability as measured through clinical balance testing. J Athl Train 2000;35:19–25.

[92] Olmsted LC, Carcia CR, Hertel J, et al. Efficacy of the Star Excursion Balance Test in detecting reach deficits in subjects with chronic ankle instability. J Athl Train 2002;37: 501–6.

[93] Gribble PA, Hertel J, Denegar CR, et al. The effects of fatigue and chronic ankle instability on dynamic postural control. J Athl Train 2004;39:321–9.

[94] Hertel J, Braham RA, Hale SA, et al. Simplifying the Star Excursion Balance Test: analyses of subjects with and without chronic ankle instability. J Orthop Sports Phys Ther 2006;36: 131–7.

[95] Hale SA, Hertel J, Olmsted-Kramer LC. Lower extremity function improves after rehabilitation for chronic ankle instability. J Orthop Sports Phys Ther 2007;37:303–11.

[96] Crosbie J, Green T, Refshauge K. Effects of reduced ankle dorsiflexion following lateral ligament sprain on temporal and spatial gait parameters. Gait Posture 1999;9:167–72.

[97] Green T, Refshauge K, Crosbie J, et al. A randomized controlled trial of a passive accessory joint mobilization on acute ankle inversion sprains. Phys Ther 2001;81:984–94.

[98] Spaulding SJ, Livingston LA, Hartsell HD. The influence of external orthotic support on the adaptive gait characteristics of individuals with chronically unstable ankles. Gait Posture 2003;17:152–8.

[99] Becker HP, Rosenbaum D, Claes L, et al. Dynamic pedography for assessing functional ankle joint instability. Unfallchirurg 1997;100:133–9.

[100] Nyska M, Shabat S, Simkin A, et al. Dynamic force distribution during level walking under the feet of patients with chronic ankle instability. Br J Sports Med 2003;37:495–7.

[101] Monaghan K, Delahunt E, Caulfield B. Ankle function during gait in patients with chronic ankle instability compared to controls. Clin Biomech 2006;21(2):168–74.

[102] Delahunt E, Monaghan K, Caulfield B. Altered neuromuscular control and ankle joint kinematics during walking in subjects with functional instability of the ankle joint. Am J Sports Med 2006;34(12):1970–6.

[103] Caulfield BM, Garrett M. Functional instability of the ankle: differences in patterns of ankle and knee movement prior to and post landing in a single leg jump. Int J Sports Med 2002;23:64–8.

[104] Caulfield B, Garrett M. Changes in ground reaction force during jump landing in subjects with functional instability of the ankle joint. Clin Biomech 2002;19:617–21.

[105] Delahunt E, Monaghan K, Caulfield B. Changes in lower limb kinematics, kinetics, and muscle activity in subjects with functional instability of the ankle joint during a single leg drop jump. J Orthop Res 2006;24(10):1991–2000.

[106] Fu SN, Hui-Chan CW. Modulation of prelanding lower-limb muscle responses in athletes with multiple ankle sprains. Med Sci Sports Exerc 2007;39(10):1774–83.

[107] Ashton-Miller JA, Wojtys EM, Huston LJ, et al. Can proprioception really be improved by exercises? Knee Surg Sports Traumatol Arthrosc 2001;9(3):128–36.

[108] Docherty CL, Moore JH, Arnold BL. Effects of strength training on strength development and joint position sense in functionally unstable ankles. J Athl Train 1998;33(4):310–4.

[109] Hopkins J, Ingersoll CD, Edwards J, et al. Cryotherapy and transcutaneous electric neuromuscular stimulation decrease arthrogenic muscle inhibition of the vastus medialis after knee joint effusion. J Athl Train 2002;37(1):25–31.

[110] Wester JU, Jespersen SM, Nielsen KD, et al. Wobble board training after partial sprains of the lateral ligaments of the ankle: a prospective randomized study. J Orthop Sports Phys Ther 1996;23:332–6.

[111] Verhagen E, van der Beek A, Twisk J, et al. The effect of a proprioceptive balance board training program for the prevention of ankle sprains. Am J Sports Med 2004;32: 1385–93.

[112] McGuine TA, Keene JS. The effect of a balance training program on risk of ankle injury in high school athletes. Am J Sports Med 2006;34:1103–11.

[113] Rozzi SL, Lephart SM, Sterner R, et al. Balance training for persons with functionally unstable ankles. J Orthop Sports Phys Ther 1999;29(8):478–86.

[114] Bernier JN, Perrin DH. Effect of coordination training on proprioception of the functionally unstable ankle. J Orthop Sports Phys Ther 1998;27(4):264–75.

[115] Taube W, Gruber M, Gollhofer A. Spinal and supraspinal adaptations associated with balance training and their functional relevance. Acta Physiol 2008 [Epub ahead of print].

[116] Ross SE. Noise-enhanced postural stability in subjects with functional ankle instability. Br J Sports Med 2007;41(10):656–9.

[117] Ross SE, Arnold BL, Blackburn JT, et al. Enhanced balance associated with coordination training with stochastic resonance stimulation in subjects with functional ankle instability: an experimental trial. J Neuroeng Rehabil 2007;4:47.

[118] Khin-Myo-Hla, Ishii T, Sakane M, et al. Effect of anesthesia of the sinus tarsi on peroneal reaction time in patients with functional instability of the ankle. Foot Ankle Int 1999;20(9):554–9.

Clin Sports Med 27 (2008) 371–382

CLINICS IN SPORTS MEDICINE

ELSEVIER
SAUNDERS

Interventions for the Prevention of First Time and Recurrent Ankle Sprains

Patrick O. McKeon, PhD, ATC, CSCS[a],*,
Carl G. Mattacola, PhD, ATC[b]

[a]Division of Athletic Training, University of Kentucky, College of Health Sciences,
Wethington Building, Room 206C, 900 South Limestone, Lexington, KY 40536-0200, USA
[b]Division of Athletic Training, University of Kentucky, College of Health Sciences,
Wethington Building, Room 210E, 900 South Limestone, Lexington, KY 40536-0200, USA

Ankle sprains are among the most common injuries in the physically active population [1–3]. It is estimated that 23,000 ankle sprains occur daily in the United States, which translates to about 1 sprain per 10,000 people every day [4]. The primary predisposing factor to suffering an ankle sprain is a history of previous sprains [5]. Although ankle sprains often are viewed as mild injuries, they represent a significant public health problem [6,7]. It has been estimated that sprains to the ankle/foot account for 1.6 million physician office visits and over 8000 hospitalizations per year [8]. Approximately 30% of those who suffer a first-time ankle sprain develop chronic ankle instability (CAI); however this rate has been reported as high as 70% [9,10]. Residual symptoms of ankle sprains can alter the health of individuals who suffer from recurrent instability significantly, causing them to become less active over the life span [11].

At the high school level, ankle sprains are the most common injury suffered out of all lower extremity injuries [12]. The highest prevalences of ankle sprains were in boys' and girls' basketball and soccer, boys' football, and girls' volleyball [13]. According to Injury Surveillance System data from the National Collegiate Athletic Association, ankle sprain was the most common injury in men's and women's basketball [14,15], men's and women's soccer [16,17], women's volleyball [18], and the second most common injury in men's football [19]. In addition, ankle injuries have been reported to be a major cause of early development of osteoarthritis [20,21]. Based on this information, ankle instability represents a major obstacle to the health and well-being of the physically active within the United States.

Although there has been considerable research on risk factors associated with ankle sprains [5], there is not a clear consensus on the most appropriate intervention strategies to prevent them. The epidemiological evaluation of risk and the identification of risk factors establish the contributing causes of this major

*Corresponding author. E-mail address: patrick.mckeon@uky.edu (P.O. McKeon).

0278-5919/08/$ – see front matter
doi:10.1016/j.csm.2008.02.004

problem. The development and implementation of prevention programs that alter identified risk factors and the systematic evaluation of the efficacy of those interventions are essential in the direction towards problem resolution [22,23].

PREVENTION OF ANKLE SPRAINS

Over the past 40 years, intervention strategies have been introduced for the prevention of first-time ankle sprains and the recurrence of ankle instability after suffering a first-time sprain. These interventions have included balance/coordination training, sport/activity-specific technical training, external support (bracing/taping), foot orthotics, footwear, and strengthening/stretching. In the past 10 years, there have been several systematic reviews that have focused on the efficacy of these strategies for treating acute [24–26] and chronic ankle instability [26,27] and their prophylactic effects in the prevention of ankle sprains [26,28]. Of all of these intervention strategies, the most consistent evidence supports the prophylactic effects of the use of external support [28,29] or balance/coordination training [26,28] in the prevention of first-time and recurrent sprains. The purpose of this article is to provide the reader with an overview of these prevention strategies, what is known in the literature, what is not known, and what is needed to be known. Throughout the manuscript, evidence will be classified according to the International Classification of Function, Disability, and Health (ICF) as activity-specific or participation-specific. In addition, guidelines will be provided based on the most current evidence to support these interventions and the goals of future research.

EXTERNAL SUPPORT AND ANKLE SPRAINS

External Support and the Prevention of Ankle Sprains

Of all the prevention strategies that have been introduced over the past 40 years, the use of external support has been shown to have the most consistent effect on the reduction in ankle sprain risk associated with physical activity [30]. These effects have been investigated in fairly diverse populations ranging from the general public, to high school athletes, collegiate athletes, professional athletes, and military recruits [25,28,29]. In a 2001 systematic review of the literature of prevention strategies for ankle sprains, Handoll and colleagues [29] found that there is clear evidence to support the use of external support such as semirigid or lace-up braces and taping for the prevention of ankle sprains. These interventions have been shown to decrease the risk of ankle sprain by 50% to 70% in those who have a history of ankle sprain. This is critical in what has been established about the prevention of ankle sprains. These interventions appear to be most effective in those who have sustained a previous ankle sprain. In those who have not sustained a previous ankle sprain, the prophylactic effects are not as clear. Therefore, providing individuals with a history of ankle sprain who participate in activities associated with a high risk of ankle sprain such as basketball, volleyball, soccer, and football appears to be a valid prophylactic measure for the prevention of recurrent sprains.

The external support of choice should be based on comfort, perceived instability, and cost [31,32]. Olmsted and colleagues [33] found that taping and bracing were equally effective at preventing ankle sprains in those who had a history of sprain among community-based soccer players and collegiate intramural basketball players. According the numbers-needed-to-treat (NNT) analysis, taping and bracing have much greater prophylactic effects for those who have a history of sprain [33]. The prophylactic effects for those without a history of sprain are negligible compared with those who have a history. This suggests that screening for those individuals who have a history of ankle sprain and providing external support would be an effective strategy for preventing future sprains. There is evidence to suggest that taping and bracing offer similar prophylactic effects in those who have a history of sprain [25,33]. The cost of taping, however, may be 3 to 25 times higher than the cost of bracing those who are at risk based on the type of activity, the number of tape applications, and number of people participating [33]. It also should be noted that semirigid stirrup braces may be applied more easily than lace-up braces because of a less complicated design [32]. This may be an important issue with regards to compliance of brace application.

Although the prophylactic effects of external support appear to be clear, there also has been concern regarding the detrimental effects of bracing on functional performance [34]. The application of ankle braces has been shown to have no significant detrimental effects on functional performance measures such as rapidly changing direction [35], sprinting [36], and vertical jump [34]. Improvements on these tasks have been found for those who have postacute or recurrent sprains [35]. Recently, the placebo effect of taping has been demonstrated in functional activities in those who have chronic ankle instability [37]. Subjects reported feeling more stable, confident, and reassured with the application of the standard taping technique (stir-ups, figure of 8, heel-lock) or a single strip of tape applied to the calf compared with the untaped condition while performing functional tasks such as hopping and balancing [33]. Although taping and bracing have been touted with providing mechanical support, it is apparent that the mechanisms for functional improvements in perceived stability remain unknown. Currently, there is no evidence to suggest that long-term brace application has detrimental effects on the functional performance in those who are already at a high level of physical activity. The long-term reliance on external support may be most appropriate for those conditions where the patient may be at a high risk for injury such as participation in cutting and jumping sports (ie, soccer, volleyball, basketball, football) or changing environmental conditions such as hiking or cross country running.

External Support and Lateral Ankle Sprain Outcomes

There have been several methods introduced for the conservative treatment of acute ankle sprains. Of these, the most effective appears to be those interventions that focus on functional treatment of the ankle rather than immobilization [24,30,38]. Immobilization as a conservative treatment strategy for acute lateral ankle sprains has been shown to have significant short- and long-term negative consequences on the function of the ankle [24,30,38]. Functional treatment includes such interventions as early mobilization and providing external support through the utilization of taping, lace-up, or semi-rigid braces. In addition, the standard rehabilitation protocol, which emphasizes the reduction of pain and swelling and the restoration of strength; range of motion, including proper arthrokinematics [39]; and balance/coordination, is part of the functional treatment progression.

Based on a review of evidence, Struijs and Kerkhoffs [30] found that functional treatment was the superior approach for reducing the sequelae of ankle sprain such as recurrent instability, pain, and significant time loss from work or sport. The role of external support played a critical role in these outcomes. The use of external support is an effective strategy for reducing the perception of joint instability and shortening the time to return to work/sport [25]. External support included the use of tape and semirigid and lace-up braces. Kerkhoffs and colleagues [25] reported no differences in the reported symptoms of pain, subjective instability, objective instability, or range of motion among these types of external supports in those who suffered lateral ankle sprain. Based on this information, it is apparent that providing external support in conjunction with functional treatments addressing pain, strength, range of motion, and balance/coordination appear to be effective in shortening the time to return to work/sport [25,31,40]. The selection of these external supports should be based on comfort, convenience of application, and cost-effectiveness [25,33,34].

Future Directions

There is a paucity of evidence to support the assumption that external support after ankle injury returns the patient to normal functional participation in the long term. The evidence is clear that the risk of ankle sprain is reduced with the application of external support over a relatively short follow-up period (up to 1 year). There is very limited to no evidence to support a change in the quality of life in these individuals. Do these individuals return to a normal level of involvement in life situations related to the application of external support? If so, it then becomes important to determine the quality of participation, the perception of disability associated with participation in work/sport, and the ability to participate at the desired skill level. In addition, it would be clinically important to know whether there are discrepancies in the amount of exposure to work/sport individuals have after ankle sprain with the use of external support compared with preinjury status. It may be that those who receive external support participate less than, more cautiously, and/or at a lower skill level than preinjury level. Those confounding factors therefore lead to a decreased incidence of recurrent sprain.

Based on what has been established in the literature, it is apparent that more well-designed, high-quality, large-scale clinical trials of bracing and taping to prevent ankle sprains are warranted [25]. These clinical trials should not only evaluate the effects of external support on variables such as time-to-return to work/sport, but also on participation-specific outcomes such as quality of life with the application of external support, level of disability associated with involvement in sport and/or work, change in status of exposure to sport or work environments, and perception of participation compared with before injury. Do these interventions significantly alter the perception of disability and allow for more normal interactions than existed prior to onset of injury. Thacker and colleagues [28] recommended that external support be used for up to 6 months after ankle sprain. What remains unknown is whether the early return to sport/work with the use of external support leads to detrimental sequelae beyond the period of 6 to 12 months after injury. These components are crucial to determine whether bracing is truly a viable option for the long term or whether there are other strategies that would offer more robust prophylactic effects with less incidence of such negative consequences as the development of post-traumatic osteoarthritis [20,21].

BALANCE/COORDINATION TRAINING
Balance/Coordination Training and the Prevention of Ankle Sprains
Balance/coordination training typically involves activities in single-limb stance that challenge the person's ability to maintain balance. A major confounding factor in the interpretation of the effects of balance training is the variety of activities and programs that have been implemented. Balance training programs have utilized balance boards [41,42], foam pads [11], dynamic hopping activities [43], and technical training [43,44]. During these activities, athletes typically maintain single limb stance and perform sport-related activities such as dribbling, passing, or shooting [41,42]. Technical training associated with volleyball also has been reported [43,44]. In these activities, players are coached about proper take-off and landing techniques during various volleyball-specific drills. All of these activities have been demonstrated to be effective in reducing the risk of ankle sprain associated with sports such as soccer, volleyball, and basketball [26,41–43] and improving the functional outcomes of those who have acute and chronic ankle instability [26,40,45–51].

McKeon and Hertel [26] conducted a systematic review of the efficacy of balance training in reducing the risk of ankle sprain. There is strong evidence from several prospective studies [41–43] that balance/coordination training is effective in reducing the risk of ankle sprains, especially in those who have a previous history of sprain [41,42]. Bahr and colleagues [43] demonstrated that the longer a prevention program with components of balance training is employed, the greater the prophylactic benefit. The balance training prevention program implemented for 2 consecutive years provided greater ankle sprain risk reduction (49%) compared with 1 year (21%) [42]. In addition, the NNT analysis revealed a shift from 27 players in the first year to 12 players in the second year in order to prevent one ankle sprain [26]. These results should be interpreted with caution considering the homogenous sample used of elite male volleyball players. McGuine and Keene [42] and Verhagen and colleagues [41] demonstrated that season-long programs performed three to five times per week that involve single limb stance balance training activities that incorporated stable and unstable surfaces as well as sport specific components such as throwing and catching a ball, dribbling, and passing were effective in reducing the incidence of ankle sprain during participation in an athletic season. Based on an NNT analysis of these studies, McKeon and Hertel [26] determined that in order to prevent one ankle sprain, an average of 26 players would need to undergo balance training in order to prevent one subsequent sprain. In those who had a history of sprain, the NNT was reduced to an average of 21.5. For those without a history of ankle sprain, the reduction in risk is less clear. It is again apparent that those who have a history of ankle sprain benefit most from balance and coordination interventions.

Balance/Coordination Training and Acute Lateral Ankle Sprain Outcomes

The performance of single-limb balance exercises on an unstable surface has shown promise as an effective intervention for reducing the recurrence of injury after acute ankle sprain [40,45]. In these studies, the use of a wobble board, balance exercises with eyes open and eyes closed, and functional activities such as figure of 8 running exercises provided significant prophylactic effects on the recurrence of ankle sprains after treatment for acute sprain [40,45]. Holme and colleagues [40] compared the outcomes after acute ankle sprain between those who received a supervised functional rehabilitation program twice a week and those who received information regarding a standard home rehabilitation protocol. Wester and colleagues [45] compared the outcomes after acute ankle sprain of those who received a 12-week home-based wobble board program with those who received only standard treatment. Both of these studies had a post-treatment follow-up period where patients were contacted to report whether a sprain had occurred after rehabilitation. Based on relative risk analysis of these studies, McKeon and Hertel [26] calculated a 54% to 76% relative risk reduction of suffering recurrent ankle sprain after undergoing these types of balance training programs following acute ankle sprain. In addition, those who underwent balance training reported fewer episodes of instability at follow up. The follow-up periods for these studies were an average of 230 days [45] to 12 months [40].

Balance/Coordination Training and Chronic Ankle Instability Outcomes

Those who suffer from chronic ankle instability also have been shown to benefit from balance training. Various programs have been introduced that involve maintaining single-limb stance on stable and unstable surfaces, performance of functional activities such as hopping and figure of 8 running, and general strengthening [46–52]. These programs have been implemented from 4 to 8 weeks for one to five times per week. Rozzi and colleagues [51], Hale and colleagues [49], and McKeon and colleagues [50] demonstrated that performing supervised balance training for 4 weeks significantly improves self-reported measures of disability in those who have chronic ankle instability. Eils and Rosenbaum [46] established that after 12 months, those with CAI who undergo balance training report a 60% decrease in episodes of the ankle giving way. Based on these studies, there appears some evidence that balance training is effective in improving the level of function in those who have CAI; yet there is no direct evidence to support a reduction in the risk of recurrent ankle sprain.

Future Directions

Throughout the literature on the effects of balance/coordination training on the outcomes of those with ankle sprain, it is unknown what types of programs offer the most benefit to those who have ankle instability, or to those who may go on to suffer a first-time sprain. It is important to establish whether a progression of low-impact activities such as the maintenance of single-limb stance on stable and unstable surfaces to more dynamic activities such as running, cutting, and hopping offer greater prophylactic benefit than programs that only rely on single-limb stance activities. The length of follow-up after balance/coordination training and the information obtained in the follow-ups are also crucial outcomes to address. Do those who undergo balance/coordination training after ankle injury report improved quality of life, less osteoarthritis, and less ankle sprains than those who do not over a follow-up period longer than 1 year? In addition, the optimal time to introduce a balance training program (eg, preseason, off-season, within the first 2 weeks after injury), the optimal length of a balance training program (eg, 4 weeks, 6 weeks, season-long), the number of sessions per week (eg, one, three, five, daily), and the length of each session (10 minutes to 1 hour) still need to be established.

CONTINUUM OF INSTABILITY: ARE WE ASSESSING DISABILITY?

There has been extensive research on the role of external support and other interventions on the perceived ankle instability a person experiences who has suffered a sprain. There is little evidence, however, that connects that local instability with global disability. In 1980, the World Health Organization developed a model in an attempt to provide standardized language for health and health-related states. This model is known as the ICF [53]. Human functioning is classified by the ICF as having three levels. These include functioning at the level of the body or body part, functioning at the level of the person as a whole, and functioning at the level of the whole person in a societal context. These functions are labeled broadly: Body functions and structure, activity, and participation, respectively [53]. Rather than viewing function and disability as separate, the ICF views these two as individual aspects as outcomes associated with the interaction between a health condition and contextual factors such as the environment. The ICF model provides a framework for the descriptions of function and disability as they relate to body structures and function, activity, and participation. Impairments refer to changes in body structure or function associated with a health condition (ie, ankle sprain). Activity is related to execution of a task (ie, running, cutting, hopping), whereas participation refers to involvement in a life situation (playing soccer). Limitations of activity refer to difficulty performing a task, and restrictions in participation refer to problems that an individual experiences when involved in life situations. The purpose of this model is to develop the framework for a common language to be used as a tool to chart the detriments of health conditions and the benefits of interventions to treat and prevent them. The physiological, neuromuscular, and biomechanical impairments associated with ankle instability have been studied extensively; however, clear evidence as to the reduction in risk based on the structural or functional modifications from the interventions discussed previously have not been well established.

Despite the evidence to support conservative functional treatment of ankle sprains, the recurrence of ankle instability after initial sprain and the propensity for developing post-traumatic osteoarthritis [20,21] are noteworthy. From the structural framework of the ICF model and the evidence presented previously, it is apparent that the application of external support and the implementation of balance training programs have a positive influence at the activity limitations and participation restrictions in those with ankle instability. The structural and functional changes associated with these improvements that occur with these interventions remain unclear.

In both intervention strategies discussed previously, those who benefit from the prophylactic effects of external support and balance training are those who have a history of a previous sprain. This indicates that those with the health condition (ankle instability) have greater prophylactic benefit than those without the health condition. Both strategies reduce the risk of ankle sprains over a relatively short follow-up period and return those who have ankle sprain back to participation in work/sport sooner than those who do not receive these interventions. There is a paucity of evidence to suggest that those who return to work/sport with the use of external support or after undergoing balance training are at less risk of developing osteoarthritis, other functional impairments associated with ankle injury, and have improved quality of life in the long term [54]. These outcomes need to be established. Several clinimetric instruments have been established to quantify the amount of disability a person experiences because of foot/ankle injury. The Foot and Ankle Disability Index [49,50,55] (now the Foot and Ankle Ability Measure [56]) and the Ankle Joint Functional Assessment Tool [51] have been used to quantify improvements in self-reported function after balance training in those who have CAI. The utilization of instruments such as these is an essential component of determining the long-term efficacy of the interventions discussed previously.

Verhagen and colleagues [57] found that those who have a history of ankle sprain within the past year are at significantly greater risk of suffering another sprain throughout a competitive volleyball season. For those who had a history of sprain who had not suffered one in over a year, however, the risk of suffering a sprain during the season was equal to those who had never suffered a sprain. This becomes critical when making decisions with regard to the length of intervention studies, the strategies to reduce the recurrence of sprains, and the follow-up period after study. Specifically, it is important when advising individuals who have suffered a sprain that proper rehabilitation and implementation of prevention strategies must be employed to reduce future occurrences of an ankle sprain.

The prescription of activity modifications over a lifetime and maintenance therapy is not understood clearly. Recommendations to perform balance training and the use of external support often are limited to the initial treatment period. It would be expected that someone with ligamentous or proprioceptive compromise from injury would need to devote attention to this limitation throughout life. Although modification of lifestyle and alterations in diet and exercise are common prescriptions by a physician to prevent heart attack or high blood pressure, this is not always the case with ankle sprains. It is known that there is a high recurrence rate, yet specific strategies for reducing injury over the long term is not common practice, and little is documented or known from clinical trials. Health care professionals may be limiting their ability to provide the best care by not providing specific rehabilitative exercise (balance training and strengthening) and suggestions for participation after patients are treated for an acute injury. For example, for patients who wish to participate in cutting activities, a maintenance program of exercises and recommendation to prophylactically brace in high-risk activities might prevent reoccurrence of ankle sprains. It is not known if a more comprehensive approach to managing acute and chronic injuries would result in a reduction of the prevalence of injuries or reduction in health care costs and days lost because of injury.

FURTHER DIRECTIONS

Based on the evidence presented, there is a need to establish long-term outcomes associated with the use of external support and balance training in those who have ankle instability. It is apparent that the use of external support decreases the time to return to work/sport after ankle sprain. What needs to be established is whether this early return with the use of external support substantially improves the quality of life and significantly reduces the risk of osteoarthritis in these patients. Balance training also appears to offer clear prophylactic effects for those with ankle instability. What needs to be established are the optimal types of activities that produce the greatest risk reduction in those who have ankle instability. Well-designed clinical trials assessing the prophylactic effects of various balance training programs are warranted. These trials must include long-term follow-up periods that address outcomes related to disability, injury recurrence, and the development of osteoarthritis. Lastly, the combination of balance training and external support needs to be investigated. Are the prophylactic benefits of implementing both interventions greater than one or the other?

SUMMARY

The use of external support and balance training individually reduces the risk of reinjury in those who have a history of ankle instability. Better assessment of outcomes associated with the ICF model through systematic study of these two interventions may provide better answers to treatment paradigms. Most importantly, the application of external support and balance training are effective in assisting patients in returning to function, especially following an acute injury.

References

[1] Fong DT, Hong Y, Chan LK, et al. A systematic review on ankle injury and ankle sprain in sports. Sports Med 2007;37(1):73–94.

[2] Almeida SA, Williams KM, Shaffer RA, et al. Epidemiological patterns of musculoskeletal injuries and physical training. Med Sci Sports Exerc 1999;31(8):1176–82.

[3] Anandacoomarasamy A, Barnsley L. Long-term outcomes of inversion ankle injuries. Br J Sports Med 2005;39(3):e1–4.

[4] Kannus P, Renstrom P. Treatment for acute tears of the lateral ligaments of the ankle. Operation, cast, or early controlled mobilization. J Bone Joint Surg Am 1991;73(2): 305–12.

[5] Beynnon BD, Murphy DF, Alosa DM. Predictive factors for lateral ankle sprains: a literature review. J Athl Train 2002;37(4):376–80.

[6] Soboroff SH, Pappius EM, Komaroff AL. Benefits, risks, and costs of alternative approaches to the evaluation and treatment of severe ankle sprain. Clin Orthop Relat Res 1984;183: 160–8.

[7] Verhagen RA, de Keizer G, van Dijk CN. Long-term follow-up of inversion trauma of the ankle. Arch Orthop Trauma Surg 1995;114(2):92–6.

[8] Praemer A, Furner S, Rice D. Musculoskeletal conditions in the United States. Rosemont (IL): American Academy of Orthopaedic Surgeons; 1999.

[9] Smith RW, Reischl SF. Treatment of ankle sprains in young athletes. Am J Sports Med 1986;14(6):465–71.

[10] Peters JW, Trevino SG, Renstrom PA. Chronic lateral ankle instability. Foot Ankle 1991;12(3):182–91.

[11] McHugh MP, Tyler TF, Mirabella MR, et al. The effectiveness of a balance training intervention in reducing the incidence of noncontact ankle sprains in high school football players. Am J Sports Med 2007;35(8):1289–94.

[12] Fernandez WG, Yard EE, Comstock RD. Epidemiology of lower extremity injuries among US high school athletes. Acad Emerg Med 2007;14(7):641–5.

[13] Nelson AJ, Collins CL, Yard EE, et al. Ankle injuries among United States high school sports athletes, 2005–2006. J Athl Train 2007;42(3):381–7.

[14] Dick R, Hertel J, Agel J, et al. Descriptive epidemiology of collegiate men's basketball injuries: National Collegiate Athletic Association Injury Surveillance System, 1988–1989 through 2003–2004. J Athl Train 2007;42(2):194–201.

[15] Agel J, Olson DE, Dick R, et al. Descriptive epidemiology of collegiate women's basketball injuries: National Collegiate Athletic Association Injury Surveillance System, 1988–1989 through 2003–2004. J Athl Train 2007;42(2):202–10.

[16] Agel J, Evans TA, Dick R, et al. Descriptive epidemiology of collegiate men's soccer injuries: National Collegiate Athletic Association Injury Surveillance System, 1988–1989 through 2002–2003. J Athl Train 2007;42(2):270–7.

[17] Dick R, Putukian M, Agel J, et al. Descriptive epidemiology of collegiate women's soccer injuries: National Collegiate Athletic Association Injury Surveillance System, 1988–1989 through 2002–2003. J Athl Train 2007;42(2):278–85.

[18] Agel J, Palmieri-Smith RM, Dick R, et al. Descriptive epidemiology of collegiate women's volleyball injuries: national Collegiate Athletic Association Injury Surveillance System, 1988–1989 through 2003–2004. J Athl Train 2007;42(2):295–302.

[19] Dick R, Ferrara MS, Agel J, et al. Descriptive epidemiology of collegiate men's football injuries: national Collegiate Athletic Association Injury Surveillance System, 1988–1989 through 2003–2004. J Athl Train 2007;42(2):221–33.

[20] Drawer S, Fuller CW. Propensity for osteoarthritis and lower limb joint pain in retired professional soccer players. Br J Sports Med 2001;35(6):402–8.

[21] Saltzman CL, Salamon ML, Blanchard GM, et al. Epidemiology of ankle arthritis: report of a consecutive series of 639 patients from a tertiary orthopaedic center. Iowa Orthop J 2005;25:44–6.

[22] Sports-related injuries among high school athletes—United States, 2005–06 school year. MMWR Morb Mortal Wkly Rep 2006;55(38):1037–40.

[23] van Mechelen W, Hlobil H, Kemper HC. Incidence, severity, aetiology, and prevention of sports injuries. A review of concepts. Sports Med 1992;14(2):82–99.

[24] Kerkhoffs GM, Rowe BH, Assendelft WJ, et al. Immobilisation and functional treatment for acute lateral ankle ligament injuries in adults. Cochrane Database Syst Rev 2002;(3): CD003762.

[25] Kerkhoffs GM, Struijs PA, Marti RK, et al. Different functional treatment strategies for acute lateral ankle ligament injuries in adults. Cochrane Database Syst Rev 2002;(3):CD002938.

[26] McKeon PO, Hertel J. Systematic review of postural control and lateral ankle instability, part 2: Is Balance Training Clinically Effective? Journal of Athletic Training, in press.

[27] deVries J, Krips R, Sierevelt I, et al. Interventions for treating chronic ankle instability. Cochrane Database Syst Rev 2006;4:CD004124.

[28] Thacker SB, Stroup DF, Branche CM, et al. The prevention of ankle sprains in sports. A systematic review of the literature. Am J Sports Med 1999;27(6):753–60.

[29] Handoll HH, Rowe BH, Quinn KM, et al. Interventions for preventing ankle ligament injuries. Cochrane Database Syst Rev 2001;(3):CD000018.

[30] Struijs P, Kerkhoffs G. Ankle sprain. Clin Evid 2006;15:1493–501.

[31] Mattacola CG, Dwyer MK. Rehabilitation of the ankle after acute sprain or chronic instability. J Athl Train 2002;37(4):413–29.

[32] Rosenbaum D, Kamps N, Bosch K, et al. The influence of external ankle braces on subjective and objective parameters of performance in a sports-related agility course. Knee Surg Sports Traumatol Arthrosc 2005;13(5):419–25.

[33] Olmsted LC, Vela LI, Denegar CR, et al. Prophylactic ankle taping and bracing: a numbers-needed-to-treat and cost-benefit analysis. J Athl Train 2004;39(1):95–100.

[34] Cordova ML, Scott BD, Ingersoll CD, et al. Effects of ankle support on lower-extremity functional performance: a meta-analysis. Med Sci Sports Exerc 2005;37(4):635–41.

[35] Jerosch J, Thorwesten L, Frebel T, et al. Influence of external stabilizing devices of the ankle on sport-specific capabilities. Knee Surg Sports Traumatol Arthrosc 1997;5(1):50–7.

[36] Hals TM, Sitler MR, Mattacola CG. Effect of a semirigid ankle stabilizer on performance in persons with functional ankle instability. J Orthop Sports Phys Ther 2000;30(9): 552–6.

[37] Sawkins K, Refshauge K, Kilbreath S, et al. The placebo effect of ankle taping in ankle instability. Med Sci Sports Exerc 2007;39(5):781–7.

[38] Kerkhoffs GM, Struijs PA, van Dijk CN. Acute treatment of inversion ankle sprains: immobilization versus functional treatment. Clin Orthop Relat Res 2007;463:250–1 [author reply 251].

[39] Denegar CR, Hertel J, Fonseca J. The effect of lateral ankle sprain on dorsiflexion range of motion, posterior talar glide, and joint laxity. J Orthop Sports Phys Ther 2002;32(4): 166–73.

[40] Holme E, Magnusson SP, Becher K, et al. The effect of supervised rehabilitation on strength, postural sway, position sense, and reinjury risk after acute ankle ligament sprain. Scand J Med Sci Sports 1999;9(2):104–9.

[41] Verhagen E, van der Beek A, Twisk J, et al. The effect of a proprioceptive balance board training program for the prevention of ankle sprains: a prospective controlled trial. Am J Sports Med 2004;32(6):1385–93.

[42] McGuine TA, Keene JS. The effect of a balance training program on the risk of ankle sprains in high school athletes. Am J Sports Med 2006;34(7):1103–11.

[43] Bahr R, Lian O, Bahr IA. A twofold reduction in the incidence of acute ankle sprains in volleyball after the introduction of an injury prevention program: a prospective cohort study. Scand J Med Sci Sports 1997;7(3):172–7.

[44] Stasinopoulos D. Comparison of three preventive methods in order to reduce the incidence of ankle inversion sprains among female volleyball players. Br J Sports Med 2004;38(2): 182–5.

[45] Wester JU, Jespersen SM, Nielsen KD, et al. Wobble board training after partial sprains of the lateral ligaments of the ankle: a prospective randomized study. J Orthop Sports Phys Ther 1996;23(5):332–6.

[46] Bernier JN, Perrin DH. Effect of coordination training on proprioception of the functionally unstable ankle. J Orthop Sports Phys Ther 1998;27(4):264–75.

[47] Eils E, Rosenbaum D. A multistation proprioceptive exercise program in patients with ankle instability. Med Sci Sports Exerc 2001;33(12):1991–8.

[48] Gauffin H, Tropp H, Odenrick P. Effect of ankle disk training on postural control in patients with functional instability of the ankle joint. Int J Sports Med 1988;9(2):141–4.

[49] Hale SA, Hertel J, Olmsted-Kramer LC. The effect of a 4-week comprehensive rehabilitation program on postural control and lower extremity function in individuals with chronic ankle instability. J Orthop Sports Phys Ther 2007;37(6):303–11.

[50] McKeon PO, Ingersoll CD, Kerrigan DC, et al. Balance training improves function and postural control in chronic ankle instability. Med Sci Sports Exerc [in review].

[51] Rozzi SL, Lephart SM, Sterner R, et al. Balance training for persons with functionally unstable ankles. J Orthop Sports Phys Ther 1999;29(8):478–86.

[52] Tropp H, Ekstrand J, Gillquist J. Factors affecting stabilometry recordings of single-limb stance. Am J Sports Med 1984;12(3):185–8.

[53] Jette AM. Toward a common language for function, disability, and health. Phys Ther 2006;86(5):726–34.

[54] Kerkhoffs GM, Handoll HH, de Bie R, et al. Surgical versus conservative treatment for acute injuries of the lateral ligament complex of the ankle in adults. Cochrane Database Syst Rev 2007;(2):CD000380.

[55] Hale SA, Hertel J. Reliability and sensitivity of the foot and ankle disability index in subjects with chronic ankle instability. J Athl Train 2005;40(1):35–40.

[56] Martin RL, Irrgang JJ, Burdett RG, et al. Evidence of validity for the foot and ankle ability measure (FAAM). Foot Ankle Int 2005;26(11):968–83.

[57] Verhagen EA, Van der Beek AJ, Bouter LM, et al. A one-season prospective cohort study of volleyball injuries. Br J Sports Med 2004;38(4):477–81.

Clin Sports Med 27 (2008) 383–404

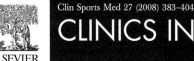

CLINICS IN SPORTS MEDICINE

LSEVIER
AUNDERS

Neuromuscular Consequences of Anterior Cruciate Ligament Injury

Christopher D. Ingersoll, PhD, ATC[a,b,*],
Terry L. Grindstaff, DPT, ATC[b,c],
Brian G. Pietrosimone, MEd, ATC[b],
Joseph M. Hart, PhD, ATC[d]

[a]Department of Human Services, University of Virginia, 210 Emmet Street South,
PO Box 4000407, Charlottesville, VA 22904, USA
[b]Exercise and Sport Injury Laboratory, University of Virginia, 210 Emmet Street South,
PO Box 400407, Charlottesville, VA 22904-4407, USA
[c]Department of Athletics, University of Virginia, Emmet and Massie Roads, PO Box 800834,
Charlottesville, VA 22904, USA
[d]Department of Orthopaedic Surgery, University of Virginia, 400 Ray C. Hunt Drive,
Suite 330, Charlottesville, VA 22908-0159, USA

The neuromuscular consequences of anterior cruciate ligament (ACL) injury are important considerations because these deficits play a crucial role in patient's recovery following ACL injury or reconstruction. The purpose of this article is to review and synthesize the known neuromuscular consequences of ACL injury and reconstruction. Specifically, changes in somatosensation, muscle activation, muscle strength, atrophy, balance, biomechanics, and patient-oriented outcomes are discussed. Understanding neuromuscular consequences aids in the construction of optimized rehabilitation strategies.

SOMATOSENSATION

The ACL and the knee joint capsule are composed of mechanoreceptors, such as free nerve endings, Ruffini endings, Golgi tendon organs, and Pacinian corpuscles, which provide information pertaining to joint position to the central nervous system for communication with the muscle [1,2]. Evidence for the physiologic connection between the ACL and the sensory cortex has been confirmed using detection of somatosensory evoked potentials following electrical stimulation of the ACL [3]. There is some controversy within the

*Corresponding author. Exercise and Sport Injury Laboratory, University of Virginia, 210 Emmet Street South, PO Box 400407, Charlottesville, VA 22904-4407. E-mail address: ingersoll@virginia.edu (C.D. Ingersoll).

0278-5919/08/$ – see front matter
doi:10.1016/j.csm.2008.03.004

literature regarding the existence of altered proprioception or somatosensory deficits in ACL-deficient (ACL-D) and ACL-reconstructed (ACL-R) patients. This controversy may be because of the wide variety of methods used to evaluate somatosensory deficits in these populations.

Active joint repositioning has been used to assess proprioceptive deficits, and generally consists of passively moving a joint to a target point in a specific range of motion and then instructing the participant to actively reposition the joint to that target position. The ability to actively reposition the knee following ACL injury has been reported to be diminished in the involved leg compared with the uninvolved leg [2–6]. Deficits in active repositioning have been reported to persist in ACL-R patients [5]. Other authors [7–10] have reported no differences in the ability to reposition injured and uninjured knee joints in ACL-D patients.

Rasmussen and Jensen [5] reported that there were significantly greater errors in ACL-D and ACL-R patients when starting at a flexed position and extending the knee compared with starting at an extended position and actively flexing the knee. Inaccuracies during active extension joint repositioning may cause increased anterior translation, which may cause inaccuracies compared with during flexion repositioning of the knee. Another study [9] performing active joint repositioning going from full extension to a flexed position has reported no difference between involved and uninvolved ACL-D, ACL-R, and control knees. Four of the five studies [2,3,5,6] reporting a decreased ability to actively reposition the injured knee were moving from a flexed position to an extended; only one study [4] reporting a decrement was moving from an extended position to a flexed position. Of the studies that reported no difference in the ability to actively reposition the injured knee, one study [7] had subjects moving from a flexed position to an extended position and four studies [5,8–10] had subjects moving from an extended position to a flexed position. Authors [8] suggested that it is possible that muscle receptors dominate afferent signaling of position during joint repositioning and compensate for altered signals from joint proprioceptors. Furthermore, it has been reported that the larger the deficit in joint position sense the worse the performance is in vertical jump measures ($r = -0.389$, $P < .05$) and one-leg hop measures ($r = -0.444$, $P < .05$) in ACL-D patients, suggesting that deficits in active joint repositioning may affect function [6].

Although actively repositioning a joint provides some information about the somatosensory system, the test is confounded by the motor component. Deficits or compensations from the central nervous system or motor neurons may not depict pure somatosensory function, but rather the function of the nervous system following contributions from sensory, central, and motor neuron deficits and compensation. Instructing the subject to passively detect the repositioned target point may be a purer measurement of proprioception. A decreased ability to passively detect joint position has been reported in ACL-D [5,11] and ACL-R patents [4,5,10] in the injured limb compared with the uninjured limb. Fischer-Rasmussen and Jensen [5] reported that ACL-D patients had a significant .21° difference between injured and involved legs, ACL-R patients had a significant .17° between legs, and there was no difference found between legs in healthy controls. The latency in which afferent signals are processed has been studied by passively moving the knee, instructing participants to identify when they first feel movement. The ability to detect passive motion of the knee has been reported to be significantly diminished in the involved leg of ACL-D patients [12–14] compared with the uninvolved leg. Friden and colleagues [14] reported a deficit in detection for movements into extension and flexion.

Somatosensory function of the lower extremity following ACL injury has been studied by electrically stimulating nerves in the lower extremity and examining impulses, termed somatosensory evoked potentials (SEP), recorded in specific zones of the sensory cortex [12,13,15]. SEPs have been reported to be altered following common peroneal nerve stimulation in patients who had damaged ACLs [15]. It has been reported that ACL-D patients displaying proprioception impairments also had altered SEPs, yet all patents who had altered SEPs did not have altered proprioception [12]. This finding may be explained by the hypothesis that altered proprioception of ACL-D knees is a chronic pathology that becomes more apparent over time [8].

MUSCLE ACTIVATION

Neuromuscular reorganization around the ACL-D or ACL-R knee may be the underlying contributing factor for other more conventionally recognized clinical impairments, such as strength loss, atrophy, and altered function. Although some researchers have examined the activation of the popliteus [16] or tibialis anterior [17] following ACL injury, most of the literature to date has focused on neuromuscular alterations in the quadriceps and hamstring muscle group. For the most part there has been a consensus among authors that a decrease in volition activation or motor unit firing exists in the quadriceps of patients who have ACL injuries [18–26].

Muscle inhibition attributable to knee joint pathology was first described by de Andrade and colleagues [27], who concluded that deformation of joint mechanoreceptors in injured knee joints relayed altered afferent information to the central nervous system, which they believed was caused by inhibition of the motor neurons of the surrounding quadriceps musculature. This phenomenon is now termed arthrogenic muscle inhibition [28] and is characterized by a reflexive decrease in motor neuron pool excitability [29], modulated by pre- and postsynaptic mechanisms [30,31], that inhibits the ability to activate the surrounding uninjured musculature following joint injury. Researchers [28,29,32] have suggested that mechanoreceptors, such as Ruffini fibers, Pacinian corpuscles, and Golgi-like endings, in the knee joint capsule or ligamentous structures of the joint are stimulated because of mechanical deformation caused by structure damage or distention of the capsule, which sends altered information to the spinal cord. Once the afferent information reaches the spinal cord it can be modulated presynaptically by GABA interneurons or postsynaptically by Renshaw cells, which are situated on motoneuron collateral fibers [30,31].

Other authors [33,34] have studied the electromyographic delay in the extensor mechanism following ACL reconstruction to determine how mechanisms other than reflexive ones previously explained might contribute to neuromuscular changes. Unfortunately there is controversy about whether an electromyographic delay in the extensor mechanism exists following ACL reconstruction. The absence of a mechanical delay has been reported and suggests that the efferent component of the neural system is not affected following ACL-R [33], whereas other authors [34] report an increased delay in an extensor response following a bone patellar bone autograft, which may be explained by increased stiffness of the extensor mechanism of alterations in the excitation coupling system.

Past researchers [35–40] have hypothesized that injury to the ACL would increase the activation of the thigh muscles to improve joint congruency and decrease shear forces at the knee joint. The ability to generate torque from the hamstrings has been hypothesized to be imperative in decreasing anterior translation of the tibia in ACL-R patients [41]. It has been hypothesized that the mechanoreceptors within the ACL and other knee ligaments transmit afferent information that may be processed as a reflex with the purpose of contracting musculature to decrease forces at the knee [42–44]. It has been reported that electrically stimulating the ACL with a train of two stimuli produced activity in the hamstring at rest [45] and inhibited the knee extensors and flexors during their respective contractions [46]. This finding provides evidence that an ACL reflex exists, and can have both an excitatory and an inhibitory component. In a study with limited subjects (three), increased activation of the hamstrings in response to a posterior perturbation has been reported in ACL-D patients, whereas healthy patients used the quadriceps to stabilize [47]. This finding provides evidence that the hamstrings are used to co-contract to respond to a perturbation.

Tsuda and colleagues [48] reported that this hamstring reflex arc was reestablished in subjects ranging from 37 to 80 months post bone patella bone autograft ACL reconstruction, suggesting that mechanoreceptor may reinnervate the grafted ACL allowing for more normalized afferent function. Reflex activity has been reported to be decreased after the ACL is anesthetized suggesting the ACL provides key information to the central nervous system about joint position sense [45]. Because of the small amount of activity that is produced in the hamstring following stimulation of the ACL, however, it has been hypothesized that this ligamentous structure is not solely responsible for sending afferent information about joint position [45]. Biedirt [49] reported that no hamstring reflex was elicited after tugging on the ACL, yet a reflex was found following a Lachman test suggesting joint receptors in structures other than the ACL are influential in producing a hamstring reflex.

The presence of altered neuromuscular control in the lower extremity has been evaluated using electromyogram (EMG) in ACL-D [16,50–55] and

ACL-R patients [19,23,41,52,56]. Some of these EMG studies have evaluated the neuromuscular alterations of the lower extremity in dynamic activities and supported the hypothesis that the hamstrings increase in activity while quadriceps activation is inhibited during landing from a jump in ACL-D patients [19].

Others reported no changes in the quadriceps but a decrease in the activation of the gastrocnemius [52]. Limbird and colleagues [57] reported that the quadriceps and gastrocnemius were inhibited while hamstrings were activated during gait. Further studies [58] have also reported that hamstring activity increases before landing, suggesting that the neuromuscular system may alter activation strategies using a feed-forward mechanism. Neuromuscular control has been reported to be altered in ACL-D patients during closed-chain activities, suggesting that altered neuromuscular control is needed to adequately perform a closed-chain task [59]. Altered neuromuscular control of the quadriceps has been termed quadriceps dyskinesia, which is an encompassing term that describes not only unwanted inhibition of the quadriceps but also inability to shut the quadriceps off during open-chain knee flexion tasks in which quadriceps tone was not needed [60].

A study by Boerboom and colleagues [51] evaluated hamstring activity in three separate groups, including copers, noncopers and healthy controls. There was no difference in hamstring activity during the stance phase of gait between copers and healthy controls, yet noncoping ACL-D patients had significantly more hamstring activity and knee flexion. Houck and colleagues [53] added that copers, noncopers, and controls used distinct activation patterns of the medial and lateral hamstrings and the vastus lateralis during unanticipated change of direction tasks during walking, which may be a possible explanation for why some ACL-D patients can cope with the injury and others cannot. Aalbersber [61] reported that ACL-D patients did not differ in the amount of quadriceps-hamstring co-contraction strategies compared with normal subjects when a shear force was applied to the knee. Ostering [56] reported less hamstring coactivation in maximal knee extension, which they attributed to an afferent denervation of the ACL following injury or reconstruction.

Central Mechanisms

Friemert and colleagues [45] concluded that the nature of the long latency (65 to 95 milliseconds) of the hamstring reflex that followed the double stimulation of the ACL suggests that the reflex is polysynaptic thus allowing central mechanisms to modulate muscle response. Other studies evaluating the motor cortex have suggested that altered function exists in ACL-injured individuals. Baumeister and colleagues [62] reported differences in cortical excitability measured by EEG during a repositioning of the ACL-R knee compared with control subjects. Other measures, such as the resting motor threshold of the motor cortex, have also been reported to be altered in the cortical hemisphere corresponding to the ACL-D knee compared with the uninvolved knee [63]. Reports of bilateral quadriceps inhibition in cases of unilateral ACL injury suggests that a crossover effect exists that most likely is caused by central nervous system mechanisms [20,26].

Gamma Motor Neuron Dysfunction

Some authors [64,65] hypothesize that although decreased sensory information caused by damaged ACL mechanoreceptors may not have a direct impact on alpha motor neuron function, alterations in afferent signals from joint receptors directly affect the gamma motor neuron system. The gamma motor system adjusts the shortening of the intrafusal fibers of the muscle spindles, regulating sensitivity, thus affecting the ability to produce a muscle contraction. Deficits in the gamma loop system of ACL-R [64,66,67] and ACL-D patients [65,68] have been reported following repetitive stimulation of the patellar tendon. Control subjects show marked decreases in quadriceps maximal voluntary contractions and EMG activity attributable to neurotransmitter depletion, heightened Ia threshold, or other presynaptic inhibitory mechanisms following repetitive vibratory stimulation. Maximal voluntary quadriceps contractions and EMG activity of ACL-injured patients remains relatively unaffected by repetitive vibratory stimulation, which suggests decreased activity in the gamma loop system. Interestingly, gamma loop dysfunction has been reported bilaterally in patients who had unilateral ACL injury, providing evidence that central nervous system mechanisms, which may be interneuronal or supraspinal in nature, may influence neuromuscular control of the entire organism following unilateral ACL injury [68]. This bilateral quadriceps gamma loop dysfunction has been reported early following reconstruction of the ACL, yet seems to resolve after approximately 18 months in the uninjured side, whereas deficits seem to persist in the injured leg [66].

Median Frequency

A decrease in median frequency has been reported in the quadriceps of the ACL-D limb [23,25,69] and when compared with healthy controls [23]. Authors [25,69] suggested that this was caused by an atrophy of type II muscle fibers.

MUSCLE STRENGTH

Quadriceps isokinetic strength deficits have been reported following ACL injury and seem to persist for patients following rehabilitation and in those who do not engage in structured rehabilitation (Table 1). Knee extension strength deficits have been reported between 6 months and 15 years postinjury in ACL-D patients who have not undergone reconstructive surgery [25,55,70–72]. Torque deficits for knee extension have been reported to vary between 10% and 38% of the torque generated in the uninjured leg [70,71,73]. When compared with matched healthy controls, quadriceps torque values have been reported bilaterally, leading some researchers [74] to suggest that torque deficit percentages relative to the uninjured leg may underestimate the true strength deficits in the injured leg following ACL injury. There is some evidence that quadriceps torque deficits in ACL-D patients decrease with time [70], indicating that there may be some ability to regain bilateral symmetry in knee extension force capabilities. Researchers [70] hypothesize that decreased

Table 1
Concentric isokinetic torque information following anterior cruciate ligament reconstruction

Author	Population	Average chronicity	Graft type	Velocity (°/s)	Quadriceps deficits (%)	Hamstring deficits (%)
Ageberg et al [95]	36 males, 20 females	15 y	—	90	5	No deficit
Anderson et al [77]	39 males, 18 females	6 mo, 1 y	22 PT, 23 HT	60	6 mo = 25, 1 y = 20	6 mo = 16, 1 y = 7
Blyth et al [96]	15 males, 15 females	2–8 y	9 PT, 21 HT	60, 180, 360	9, 6, 4	+1, +1, +6
Bryant et al 2008 [78]	9 males, 4 females	6–9 mo	PT	180	30	Not reported
Carter and Edinger [145]	106 patients	6 mo	38 PT, 68 HT	18, 300	No deficit	No deficit
De Jong et al [79]	191 patents	6 mo, 9 mo, 1 y	HT	60, 180	6 mo (36, 25), 9 mo (25, 18), 1 y (19, 16)	No deficit
Grossman et al [80]	22 males, 7 females	~16 y	22 PT, 3 HT, 3 Gortex	180, 240	12, 18	12, 12
Hiemstra et al [74]	9 males, 7 females	>1 y	8 PT, 16 HT	50–250	25	17
Hiemstra et al [81]	12 subjects	<1 y	HT	20–250	24.8	26.8
Jarvela et al [82]	65 males, 21 females	5–9 y	PT	60, 18, 240	10.3, 4.5, 5.2	0, 0, 2.9
Keays et al [83]	22 males, 9 females	33 mo	HT	60, 100	7.3, 7.8	10, 9.9
Kobayashi et al [84]	11 males, 25 females	6 mo, 1 y, 2 y	PT	60, 180	6 mo = 37, 31 1 y = 27, 18 2 y = 11, 9	6 mo = 10, 10 1 y = no deficit 2 y = no deficit
Makihara et al [97]	3 males, 13 females	26 mo	HT	60	Not reported	6%
Konishi et al [85]	39 males, 31 females	<1 y	HT	60, 180	9, 8	Not reported
Lee et al [86]	58 males, 9 females	6 mo, 1 y, 2 y	Quadriceps tendon	60, 180	6 mo = 36, 26 1 y = 18, 18 2 y = 18, 11	Not reported
Mattacola et al [87]	11 males, 9 females	1.5 y	PT	120, 240	16, 9	6, 5
Moisala et al [88]	39 males, 9 females	5 y, 9 mo	PT	60, 180	PT (10, 5) HT (7, 2)	PT (1, +1) HT (3, 0)
Nakamura et al [89]	36 males, 40 females	2 y	HT	60, 180	15, 11	8, 13
Nyland et al [90]	7 males, 11 females	2 y	Tibialis anterior	60	11	+7
Østerås et al [91]	90 subjects	6 mo	PT	60, 240	28.7, 21	3.1, 1
Segawa et al [92]	34 males, 28 females	1 y	HT	60	7	2
Seto et al [93]	19 males, 6 females	~10 y	Not reported	120, 240	33, 41	15, 16

Abbreviations: HT, hamstring tendon; PT, patellar tendon.

ability to produce quadriceps torque in ACL-D patients exists to decrease anterior shear forces at the knee. Others [40] have suggested that the hamstring muscles alter their function to assist in stabilizing the knee joint in the presence of an ACL ligamentous insufficiency.

Although knee flexion torques have also been reported to be diminish in ACL-D patients [70], the affect of ACL injury on the hamstring muscle group does not seem to be as devastating as reported in the quadriceps. Knee flexion torque deficits in ACL-D patients have been reported between 2% and 15% of the uninjured knee [70,71]. It has been hypothesized that the hamstrings play an important role in stabilizing the knee following ACL injury, and it has been suggested that hamstring strength may be an important factor in determining ACL-D patient function level [75]. The hamstring muscle group plays an important role during athletics and in activities of daily living, eccentrically contracting allowing for controlled deceleration and proper force attenuation. Hamstring torque deficits have been reported to practically double when assessed eccentrically (15%) compared with concentrically (8%), which may be because of altered muscle recruitment patterns that could increase the risk for subsequent injury [71].

Deficits in quadriceps strength following ACL-R have been reported at various speeds and years post-reconstruction [23,74,76–94]. Although the largest quadriceps strength deficits are reported in the first 6 to 12 months following surgery [77,84,86], deficits of between 5% and 18% of the uninvolved limb have been reported between 5 and 15 years following ACL reconstruction and extensive rehabilitation [80,88,93,95]. These quadriceps strength deficits following ACL- R are reported to be to some extent bilateral when compared with healthy matched controls. Quadriceps avoidance gait patterns and decreased ability to absorb shock during stance have been suggested to be possible risk factors to chronic joint pathologies following ACL injury.

Data regarding the effect of hamstring strength following ACL-R are not as conclusive as those concerning quadriceps strength. Some authors have reported increased hamstring deficits compared with the quadriceps following ALC-R [81,83], whereas others identify the quadriceps as having deficits that far exceed those of the hamstrings [77,82,88,91,96,97]. The controversy surrounding the amount of hamstring weakness following ACL-R may be related to graft used in the reconstruction. There has been some evidence emerging that hamstring weakness may be more associated with semitendinosus or gracilis grafts compared with bone patella bone grafts [74,88,98]. A recent study by Nyland and colleagues [90] used tibialis anterior tendon grafts, which may be the best representation of pure arthrogenic muscle inhibition following ACL-R because strength results were not confounded by tendon damage at the donor site. Nyland and colleagues [90] reported an 11% decrease in quadriceps strength and a 7% increase in hamstring strength, which may indicate altered neuromuscular control strategies present in an ACL reconstructed knee.

Although many studies [74,77,81,89,90,92] have reported strength deficits 1 to 2 years following reconstruction, little research [80,95] has determined long-term strength outcomes with modern reconstructive procedures.

ATROPHY

Muscular atrophy in the thigh muscles and legs of ACL-R and ACL-D patients is concerning because of the potential effects on the force-producing capabilities of the atrophied muscles. Quadriceps atrophy has been documented for ACL-D [72] and ACL-R [99,100] patients. The vastus medialis of ACL-D patients demonstrates decreased glycolytic activity and a shift toward more oxidative metabolism, a possible sign of active compensation for knee instability [101]. Noncopers demonstrate significantly greater quadriceps atrophy than copers [102]. Further, harvesting the semitendinosus tendon for ACL-R results in atrophy and shortening of the semitendinosus [103–105].

Adaptations in other muscles to compensate for atrophy and lost force-producing capabilities are also concerns. For example, noncopers have larger tibialis anterior muscles in the injured leg compared with the uninjured leg, possibly because of altered gait patterns in noncopers [17].

Atrophy can be prevented or become less apparent with eccentric exercise, particularly in the quadriceps and gluteus maximus muscles [106], with protein supplementation [107], or electrical stimulation [108]. Interestingly, vascular occlusion may also diminish postoperative disuse atrophy, possibly because of hormonal secretions triggered by the vascular occlusion [109].

BALANCE

The ability to maintain one's posture has been closely linked to proprioception and neuromuscular control strategies. Postural control or balance measurements have been assessed in ACL-D patients and ACL-R patients with various evaluation techniques. There is a consensus within the literature that no difference in balance exists during double-leg stance among ACL-D and ACL-R patients compared with healthy controls. Lysholm and colleagues [110] reported a significant deficit in postural control during single-leg stance with both eyes open and closed in unilateral ACL-D patients compared with healthy controls. Lysholm and colleagues [110] reported that differences were not present between injured and uninjured legs, suggesting that a bilateral deficit compared with controls was present in this group of ACL-D patients.

There is evidence that suggests a decrease in postural control measurements during closed-eye trials compared with eyes-open trials and single-leg compared with double-leg stance trials for ACL-injured patients and healthy controls [111]. In contrast to Lysholm and colleagues [110] other authors have reported no evidence of deficits in static measures of postural control among ACL-D [111,112] and ACL-R patients [87,113,114] when compared with healthy controls. Tecco and colleagues [112] reported that although no difference was found in center of pressure movement between healthy and ACL-D patients during static measures, a difference in location of center of pressure relative to the foot was found between the patient and healthy groups. The ACL-D patients were reported to encompass more anterior and medially positioned center of pressure before the commencement of static balance trials compared with the healthy controls [112]. Although an altered positioning of the center of pressure did not affect static balance trials it may be suboptimal positioning for maintaining posture following a perturbation.

There is more of a consensus among authors that the ability to maintain balance following a perturbation differs between healthy subjects and ACL-D and ACL-R patients [110,113,114]. Lysholm and colleagues [110] reported that reaction time to a perturbation was longer in ACL- D patients compared with the healthy subjects and that the injured leg had a longer reaction time compared with the uninjured leg on the healthy subjects. Henriksson and colleagues [114] also reported differences in sagittal plane ground reaction forces between ACL-R patients and healthy subjects following a perturbation, yet no differences were reported in the frontal plane. It has been stated that balance measures following a perturbation may be a better indicator of function compared with static measures because they better represent demands placed on the neuromuscular systems during functional activities [111]. Impaired balance has been hypothesized to be caused by decreased or altered mechanoreceptor information regarding joint position [113] from the injured knee, possibly resulting in modified neuromuscular control while attempting to maintain balance.

BIOMECHANICS

Following ACL injury and reconstruction changes in lower extremity kinematics, kinetics, and temporal variables have been shown to occur. Biomechanical changes in gait (walking, jogging, running), stair ambulation, and jumping have been researched extensively, but have inconsistent findings. This inconsistency may be attributed to methodologic differences between studies and the use of heterogeneous populations. Individuals who are ACL-D can be categorized into two groups, based on clinical criteria, as copers and noncopers [115,116]. Most ACL-deficient individuals fall into the classification of noncoper and experience knee instability after injury, which requires surgical reconstruction [75]. Conversely, copers are ACL-D individuals who use compensatory stabilization strategies and do not experience episodes of "giving way." These individuals have movement strategies that resemble individuals who do not have lower extremity pathology.

Biomechanical compensatory strategies are believed to be task dependent with more difficult tasks accentuating the adaptation [115,117]. Although tasks such as walking, jogging, running, stair ambulation, and jumping have similarity there are also distinct differences in muscle activation, kinematics, and kinetics. Performance on these tasks also depends on time elapsed since injury and surgical reconstruction [118,119]. Surgical reconstruction and rehabilitation have been shown to influence biomechanical adaptations and restore movement patterns that are similar to uninjured subjects [19,52,118].

Gait
Walking
There is discrepancy regarding temporal-spatial parameters of gait during walking. Earlier studies indicated that individuals who are ACL-D walk with symmetric gait pattern and with changes occurring in both the involved and uninvolved limbs [120]. Based on this finding it was suggested that the uninvolved limb not be used as a valid comparison of normal gait biomechanics [120]. More recent studies have indicated that the uninvolved limb may not have compensatory changes to the same degree as the involved limb. Step length and walking base have been shown to be smaller for the ACL-D limb compared with the uninvolved limb when comparing within the same subjects [118,119]. Based on this finding it was suggested that the uninvolved limb not be used as a valid comparison of normal gait biomechanics [120]. When comparing between healthy individuals, copers, and noncopers, step length, cadence, swing time, and stance time have been shown to be more similar [115,121]. Following surgical intervention and 4 months of rehabilitation, step length and walking base values are not significantly different from healthy individuals [118,119].

Walking electromyography. ACL-D individuals tend to stabilize the knee by using a co-contraction of the quadriceps and hamstring muscles [121,122]. Higher hamstring activity is present in the involved limb from initial contact to midstance [121,122]. Noncopers also have an earlier onset of medial gastrocnemius and a longer total duration when compared with copers and healthy controls [117]. Controversy exists regarding the presence of "quadriceps avoidance" [120,123] or decreased quadriceps activity during gait [115,118,124]. At initial contact decreased quadriceps activity may be present, but at midstance quadriceps activity between limbs is similar [122]. Decreased quadriceps activity at initial contact is coupled with higher soleus activation on the involved side [117], which may act as a secondary knee extensor by directing the tibia posteriorly when the foot is in contact with the ground [125]. At midstance the magnitude of soleus activity was lower compared with the uninvolved limb, whereas quadriceps activity was similar between limbs [122]. The compensation of the soleus is not likely needed at midstance. Eight months following ACL-R normal muscle EMG patterns of the lower extremity have been shown to return [118].

Walking kinematics. Noncopers have less knee flexion at initial contact compared with copers [115,117,121] and healthy controls [117]. Joint angles for the hip and ankle are similar for the three groups [115,121]. When comparing injured to uninjured limbs the knee flexion angle at initial contact is similar, but the involved knee has more flexion at midstance [122]. Copers use greater knee flexion during walking than noncopers and healthy controls [121]. Following surgical intervention and 4 months of rehabilitation, knee flexion angles are not similar to those of healthy individuals [118].

Walking kinetics. During the loading phase of walking individuals who have ACL-D knees demonstrate decreased knee moments that resist knee flexion [117,120] and have lower peak ground reaction force [115,117]. This pattern continues through the midstance of gait on the involved limb [122] and is believed to reduce the stress placed through the knee joint and decrease anterior tibia translation [120,126]. Load from decreased knee moments at initial contact coexists with increased contribution of hip moments [120,122]. At midstance there is a shift from greater hip moments to increased ankle moments [122]. Noncopers are believed to demonstrate the greatest decrease in knee moments [117,121] and increased hip joint moments when compared with copers and healthy controls [117].

Jogging/running
In general, jogging/running tends to exaggerate gait abnormalities compared with walking [19,52,115,117]. Compared with healthy subjects individuals who are ACL-D (copers and noncopers) have decreased jogging speed and stride length [117]. Jogging speed is slightly greater for copers when compared with noncopers, but is not significantly different [115]. Following surgical reconstruction and rehabilitation individuals tend to begin to have jogging and running biomechanics that resemble those of healthy individuals [19,52].

Jogging/running electromyography. Individuals who are ACL-D have higher hamstring EMG activity without a decrease in quadriceps EMG activity compared with individuals who have ACL reconstructions or healthy knees [19,117]. Noncopers have higher hamstring EMG activity than copers [117]. The magnitude of the differences between groups tends to be diminished during a more difficult task, such as jogging compared with walking [117].

Jogging/running kinematics. When examining a heterogeneous ACL-deficient population the amount of knee flexion during jogging was the same as healthy subjects [120]. Further examination while classifying individuals as noncopers indicated they typically limit knee joint flexion at initial contact and during the stance phase of jogging [115,117]. Copers have knee joint angles that are symmetric between sides during jogging [115]. Kinematics at the ankle do not differ between copers and noncopers [115].

Jogging/running kinetics. Noncopers have decreased knee moments at peak knee flexion on the involved limb [115,117] and decreased vertical ground reaction force during jogging compared with copers [115]. ACL-D individuals demonstrate decreased peak knee flexion moment at midstance compared with healthy subjects [120]. The hip moments increased and ankle moments remained the same and were comparable to findings during walking [117]. Loading patterns were symmetric during jogging for copers [115,120], but differed between sides for noncopers [115].

Stair Climbing
There is little difference in range of motion and forces through the lower extremity when going up and down stairs when comparing healthy subjects

and ACL-D subjects [120]. When examining noncopers, they use less knee flexion in the involved limb when ascending stairs compared with copers [115]. Noncopers also have decreased peak vertical ground reaction force compared with copers [115]. Both groups flex their involved knee less during stair descent [115].

ACL-R individuals demonstrated decreased knee extension moment during a lateral step-up task compared with healthy subjects [127]. Summated extensor moments (hip + knee + ankle) were equal to the contralateral limb or comparable to healthy values [127]. The relative contribution of each individual segment may be varied in the presence of pathology, but the sum is likely to be the same [127]. This finding indicates that although the knee extensor moment is decreased in ACL-R individuals, there is a relative increase in hip and ankle extensor moments [127].

Vertical Jump

Compared with healthy individuals, ACL-R individuals demonstrated decreased knee extension moments during vertical jump takeoff and landing [127]. Subjects also demonstrated decreased summated extensor moments (hip + knee + ankle) during vertical jump landing [127]. Summated extensors moments were not significantly different between groups for vertical jump takeoff, but were significantly different for the landing portion of the vertical jump. This finding would indicate that although the summated extensors moments were equal, the extensor moments of the hip and ankle were increased to compensate for the decreased knee extensor moment to preserve function of the lower extremity [127]. This observation was similar to findings during the step-up task. Forces during landing place the most stress on the system and that is why this task demonstrates the greatest differences [127].

FUNCTION

Instruments commonly used to assess subjective outcomes in people who have knee injury are numerous. The International Knee Documentation Committee (IKDC) subjective evaluation form was developed and validated as a "knee specific" outcomes instrument that was designed to "detect improvement or deterioration in symptoms, function and sports activity in persons with knee injury" [128–131]. Although this instrument was designed as an outcomes instrument for general knee injuries, it has been used extensively in clinical research in ACL-D and ACL-R populations. The most widely accepted scoring convention for the IKDC subjective knee evaluation form includes a normalized sum of response scored [128–131], wherein a score of 100 indicates the patient perceives no limits to function. Greater perceived limitations to function are indicated by reduced score. In retrospective study designs, a score greater than 70 can be interpreted as a successful subjective outcome; however, the scale is most effective as it is responsive to changes in perceived function over time. Other common outcomes instruments that have been used to track outcomes in knee-injured populations include the Lysholm knee scale [132], the knee disorders subjective history [133], and the Cincinnati knee score [134]. Because of the high prevalence of osteoarthritis in the ACL-injured and -reconstructed population, the Western Ontario and McMaster Universities Osteoarthritis index (WOMAC) [135] may be used in mid- and long-term outcomes studies in this population. Because ACL reconstructions are most common in young and active populations, self-reported activity rating instruments, such as the Tegner activity scale [132], are commonly used in ACL outcomes research. Finally, an extension of the WOMAC was created to evaluate short- and long-term subjective outcomes, including symptoms and function in young, physically active patients who had knee injury and osteoarthritis [136].

Recent clinical studies reporting only subjective outcomes are rare; however, subjective instrument use is ubiquitous in orthopaedic outcomes research and is typically presented descriptively or as comparisons between treatment groups or over time. Several recent studies have reported excellent subjective outcomes in ACL-R [137–139] and ACL-D [66,140] patients in the short term (2 years) [141] and mid term (5–15 years) [66,137,140]. Although ACL-R and ACL-D individuals seem to report similar levels of postinjury outcomes, people who have ACL-D knees may be achieving optimal outcomes by modifying or reducing their activity levels [66]. Although it is certainly possible for the ACL-D knee to participate in a preinjury level of activity or sport, meniscus or cartilage injury may be likely [142]. There does not seem to be a gender bias in subjective outcomes following ACL-R [143,144]; however, females may exhibit slightly greater knee laxity during clinical examination [143]. Overall, it is possible to achieve excellent outcomes and maintain a healthy and active lifestyle following ACL injury or reconstruction and there does not seem to be a difference between various graft choices or between males and females. Achieving optimal perceived outcomes and patient satisfaction remains paramount in the continuum of care for the injured athlete. Heightened risk for long-term injury and knee joint degeneration, which certainly reduces subjective outcomes, may involve neuromuscular factors that go unnoticed in the short and mid term.

SUMMARY

ACL injury and surgical reconstruction have been shown to alter lower extremity kinematics, kinetics, and temporal variables during gait. The compensatory strategy is believed to be task dependent with more difficult tasks accentuating adaptations [115,117]. Biomechanical adaptations are influenced by the time elapsed since injury [118,119] and can return to a pattern similar to uninjured subjects following surgical reconstruction and rehabilitation [19,52,118].

ACL injury seems to affect lower extremity performance during functional activities and gait. Alterations in strength may be attributable to dramatic changes in muscle activation strategies of the lower extremity, particularly the inhibition of the quadriceps and activation of the hamstring muscle groups. Although altered motor patterns may be a protective mechanism following injury, evidence suggests they persist long after ACL-R, suggesting that neuromuscular function needs to be addressed during rehabilitation.

Functional outcomes following ACL-R are generally excellent; however, persistent somatosensory and neuromuscular deficits and possible biomechanical aberrations may help explain why ACL-injured people are likely to experience early-onset knee joint osteoarthritis.

References

[1] Zimny M. Mechanoreceptors in articular cartilage. Am J Anat 1988;182:16–32.

[2] Adachi N, Ochi M, Uchio Y, et al. Mechanoreceptors in the anterior cruciate ligament contribute to the joint position sense. Acta Orthop Scand 2002;73(3):330–4.

[3] Ochi M, Iwasa J, Uchio Y, et al. Induction of somatosensory evoked potentials by mechanical stimulation in reconstructed anterior cruciate ligaments. J Bone Joint Surg Br 2002; 84(5):761–6.

[4] Bonfim TR, Jansen Paccola CA, Barela JA. Proprioceptive and behavior impairments in individuals with anterior cruciate ligament reconstructed knees. Arch Phys Med Rehabil 2003;84(8):1217–23.

[5] Fischer-Rasmussen T, Jensen PE. Proprioceptive sensitivity and performance in anterior cruciate ligament-deficient knee joints. Scand J Med Sci Sports 2000;10(2):85–9.

[6] Katayama M, Higuchi H, Kimura M, et al. Proprioception and performance after anterior cruciate ligament rupture. Int Orthop 2004;28(5):278–81.

[7] Fonseca ST, Ocarino JM, Silva PL, et al. Proprioception in individuals with ACL-deficient knee and good muscular and functional performance. Res Sports Med 2005;13(1): 47–61.

[8] Good L, Roos H, Gottlieb D, et al. Joint position sense is not changed after acute disruption of the anterior cruciate ligament. Acta Orthop Scand 1999;70(2):194–8.

[9] Reider B, Arcand MA, Diehl LH, et al. Proprioception of the knee before and after anterior cruciate ligament reconstruction. Arthroscopy 2003;19(1):2–12.

[10] Ozenci AM, Inanmaz E, Ozcanli H, et al. Proprioceptive comparison of allograft and autograft anterior cruciate ligament reconstructions. Knee Surg Sports Traumatol Arthrosc 2007;15(12):1432–7.

[11] Barrack RL, Skinner HB, Buckley SL. Proprioception in the anterior cruciate deficient knee. Am J Sports Med 1989;17(1):1–6.

[12] Courtney C, Rine RM, Kroll P. Central somatosensory changes and altered muscle synergies in subjects with anterior cruciate ligament deficiency. Gait Posture 2005; 22(1):69–74.

[13] Courtney CA, Rine RM. Central somatosensory changes associated with improved dynamic balance in subjects with anterior cruciate ligament deficiency. Gait Posture 2006;24(2):190–5.

[14] Friden T, Roberts D, Zatterstrom R, et al. Proprioception after an acute knee ligament injury: a longitudinal study on 16 consecutive patients. J Orthop Res 1997;15(5): 637–44.

[15] Valeriani M, Restuccia D, DiLazzaro V, et al. Central nervous system modifications in patients with lesion of the anterior cruciate ligament of the knee. Brain 1996;119(Pt 5): 1751–62.

[16] Weresh MJ, Gabel RH, Brand RA, et al. Popliteus function in ACL-deficient patients. Scand J Med Sci Sports 1997;7(1):14–9.

[17] Binder-Macleod BI, Buchanan TS. Tibialis anterior volumes and areas in ACL-injured limbs compared with unimpaired. Med Sci Sports Exerc 2006;38(9):1553–7.

[18] Snyder-Mackler L, De Luca PF, Williams PR, et al. Reflex inhibition of the quadriceps femoris muscle after injury or reconstruction of the anterior cruciate ligament. J Bone Joint Surg Am 1994;76(4):555–60.

[19] Swanik CB, Lephart SM, Giraldo JL, et al. Reactive muscle firing of anterior cruciate ligament-injured females during functional activities. J Athl Train 1999;34(2):121–9.

[20] Chmielewski TL, Stackhouse S, Axe MJ, et al. A prospective analysis of incidence and severity of quadriceps inhibition in a consecutive sample of 100 patients with complete acute anterior cruciate ligament rupture. J Orthop Res 2004;22(5):925–30.

[21] Urbach D, Nebelung W, Becker R, et al. Effects of reconstruction of the anterior cruciate ligament on voluntary activation of quadriceps femoris a prospective twitch interpolation study. J Bone Joint Surg Br 2001;83(8):1104–10.

[22] Urbach D, Awiszus F. Impaired ability of voluntary quadriceps activation bilaterally interferes with function testing after knee injuries. A twitch interpolation study. Int J Sports Med 2002;23(4):231–6.

[23] Drechsler WI, Cramp MC, Scott OM. Changes in muscle strength and EMG median frequency after anterior cruciate ligament reconstruction. Eur J Appl Physiol 2006; 98(6):613–23.

[24] Maitland ME, Ajemian SV, Suter E. Quadriceps femoris and hamstring muscle function in a person with an unstable knee. Phys Ther 1999;79(1):66–75.

[25] McHugh MP, Tyler TF, Nicholas SJ, et al. Electromyographic analysis of quadriceps fatigue after anterior cruciate ligament reconstruction. J Orthop Sports Phys Ther 2001;31(1): 25–32.

[26] Urbach D, Nebelung W, Weiler HT, et al. Bilateral deficit of voluntary quadriceps muscle activation after unilateral ACL tear. Med Sci Sports Exerc 1999;31(12):1691–6.

[27] de Andrade J, Grant C, Dixon A. Joint distension and reflex muscle inhibition in the knee. J Bone Joint Surg Am 1965;47(2):313–22.

[28] Hopkins J, Ingersoll C. Arthrogenic muscle inhibition: a limiting factor in joint rehabilitation. J Sport Rehabil 2000;9:135–59.

[29] Hopkins J, Ingersoll C, Krause B, et al. Effect of knee joint effusion on quadriceps and soleus motoneuron pool excitability. Med Sci Sports Exerc 2001;33(1):123–6.

[30] Palmieri R, Weltman A, Edwards J, et al. Pre-synaptic modulation of quadriceps arthrogenic muscle inhibition. Knee Surg Sports Traumatol Arthrosc 2005;13:370–6.

[31] Palmieri RM, Tom JA, Edwards JE, et al. Arthrogenic muscle response induced by an experimental knee joint effusion is mediated by pre- and post-synaptic spinal mechanisms. J Electromyogr Kinesiol 2004;14(6):631–40.

[32] Hopkins J, Ingersoll C, Edwards D, et al. Changes in soleus motorneuron pool excitability after artificial knee joint effusion. Arch Phys Med Rehabil 2000;81(9):1199–203.

[33] Georgoulis AD, Ristanis S, Papadonikolakis A, et al. Electromechanical delay of the knee extensor muscles is not altered after harvesting the patellar tendon as a graft for ACL reconstruction: implications for sports performance. Knee Surg Sports Traumatol Arthrosc 2005;13(6):437–43.

[34] Kaneko F, Onari K, Kawaguchi K, et al. Electromechanical delay after ACL reconstruction: an innovative method for investigating central and peripheral contributions. J Orthop Sports Phys Ther 2002;32(4):158–65.

[35] Johansson H, Sjolander P, Sojka P. Activity in receptor afferents from the anterior cruciate ligament evokes reflex effects on fusimotor neurones. Neurosci Res 1990;8(1):54–9.

[36] Raunest J, Sager M, Burgener E. Proprioceptive mechanisms in the cruciate ligaments: an electromyographic study on reflex activity in the thigh muscles. J Trauma 1996;41(3): 488–93.

[37] Solomonow M, Baratta R, Zhou BH, et al. The synergistic action of the anterior cruciate ligament and thigh muscles in maintaining joint stability. Am J Sports Med 1987;15(3): 207–13.

[38] Liu W, Maitland ME. The effect of hamstring muscle compensation for anterior laxity in the ACL-deficient knee during gait. J Biomech 2000;33(7):871–9.

[39] Tibone JE, Antich TJ. Electromyographic analysis of the anterior cruciate ligament-deficient knee. Clin Orthop Relat Res Mar 1993;288:35–9.

[40] Yanagawa T, Shelburne K, Serpas F, et al. Effect of hamstrings muscle action on stability of the ACL-deficient knee in isokinetic extension exercise. Clin Biomech (Bristol, Avon) 2002;17(9–10):705–12.

[41] Isaac DL, Beard DJ, Price AJ, et al. In-vivo sagittal plane knee kinematics: ACL intact, deficient and reconstructed knees. Knee 2005;12(1):25–31.

[42] Krogsgaard MR, Dyhre-Poulsen P, Fischer-Rasmussen T. Cruciate ligament reflexes. J Electromyogr Kinesiol 2002;12(3):177–82.

[43] Solomonow M. Sensory-motor control of ligaments and associated neuromuscular disorders. J Electromyogr Kinesiol 2006;16(6):549–67.

[44] Miyatsu M, Atsuta Y, Watakabe M. The physiology of mechanoreceptors in the anterior cruciate ligament. An experimental study in decerebrate-spinalised animals. J Bone Joint Surg Br 1993;75(4):653–7.

[45] Friemert B, Faist M, Spengler C, et al. Intraoperative direct mechanical stimulation of the anterior cruciate ligament elicits short- and medium-latency hamstring reflexes. J Neurophysiol 2005;94(6):3996–4001.

[46] Dyhre-Poulsen P, Krogsgaard MR. Muscular reflexes elicited by electrical stimulation of the anterior cruciate ligament in humans. J Appl Physiol 2000;89:2191–5.

[47] Di Fabio RP, Graf B, Badke MB, et al. Effect of knee joint laxity on long-loop postural reflexes: evidence for a human capsular-hamstring reflex. Exp Brain Res 1992;90(1): 189–200.

[48] Tsuda E, Ishibashi Y, Okamura Y, et al. Restoration of anterior cruciate ligament-hamstring reflex arc after anterior cruciate ligament reconstruction. Knee Surg Sports Traumatol Arthrosc 2003;11(2):63–7.

[49] Biedert RM, Zwick EB. Ligament-muscle reflex arc after anterior cruciate ligament reconstruction: electromyographic evaluation. Arch Orthop Trauma Surg 1998;118 (1–2):81–4.

[50] Kalund S, Sinkjaer T, Arendt-Nielsen L, et al. Altered timing of hamstring muscle action in anterior cruciate ligament deficient patients. Am J Sports Med 1990;18(3):245–8.

[51] Boerboom AL, Hof AL, Halbertsma JP, et al. Atypical hamstrings electromyographic activity as a compensatory mechanism in anterior cruciate ligament deficiency. Knee Surg Sports Traumatol Arthrosc 2001;9(4):211–6.

[52] Demont RG, Lephart SM, Giraldo JL, et al. Muscle preactivity of anterior cruciate ligament-deficient and -reconstructed females during functional activities. J Athl Train 1999;34(2): 115–20.

[53] Houck JR, Wilding GE, Gupta R, et al. Analysis of EMG patterns of control subjects and subjects with ACL deficiency during an unanticipated walking cut task. Gait Posture 2007;25(4):628–38.

[54] Kvist J. Sagittal tibial translation during exercises in the anterior cruciate ligament-deficient knee. Scand J Med Sci Sports 2005;15(3):148–58.

[55] Kvist J, Karlberg C, Gerdle B, et al. Anterior tibial translation during different isokinetic quadriceps torque in anterior cruciate ligament deficient and nonimpaired individuals. J Orthop Sports Phys Ther 2001;31(1):4–15.

[56] Osternig LR, Caster BL, James CR. Contralateral hamstring (biceps femoris) coactivation patterns and anterior cruciate ligament dysfunction. Med Sci Sports Exerc 1995;27(6): 805–8.

[57] Limbird TJ, Shiavi R, Frazer M, et al. EMG profiles of knee joint musculature during walking: changes induced by anterior cruciate ligament deficiency. J Orthop Res 1988;6(5): 630–8.

[58] Swanik CB, Lephart SM, Swanik KA, et al. Neuromuscular dynamic restraint in women with anterior cruciate ligament injuries. Clin Orthop Relat Res 2004;425: 189–99.

[59] Heller BM, Pincivero DM. The effects of ACL injury on lower extremity activation during closed kinetic chain exercise. J Sports Med Phys Fitness 2003;43(2):180–8.

[60] Williams GN, Barrance PJ, Snyder-Mackler L, et al. Altered quadriceps control in people with anterior cruciate ligament deficiency. Med Sci Sports Exerc 2004;36(7):1089–97.

[61] Aalbersberg S, Kingma I, Blankevoort L, et al. Co-contraction during static and dynamic knee extensions in ACL deficient subjects. J Electromyogr Kinesiol 2005;15(4):349–57.

[62] Baumeister J, Reinecke K, Weiss M. Changed cortical activity after anterior cruciate ligament reconstruction in a joint position paradigm: an EEG study. Scand J Med Sci Sports Dec 7 2007 [Epub ahead of print].

[63] Heroux ME, Tremblay F. Corticomotor excitability associated with unilateral knee dysfunction secondary to anterior cruciate ligament injury. Knee Surg Sports Traumatol Arthrosc 2006;14(9):823–33.

[64] Konishi Y, Fukubayashi T, Takeshita D. Mechanism of quadriceps femoris muscle weakness in patients with anterior cruciate ligament reconstruction. Scand J Med Sci Sports 2002;12(6):371–5.

[65] Konishi Y, Fukubayashi T, Takeshita D. Possible mechanism of quadriceps femoris weakness in patients with ruptured anterior cruciate ligament. Med Sci Sports Exerc 2002;34(9):1414–8.

[66] Kostogiannis I, Ageberg E, Neuman P, et al. Activity level and subjective knee function 15 years after anterior cruciate ligament injury: a prospective, longitudinal study of nonreconstructed patients. Am J Sports Med 2007;35(7):1135–43.

[67] Richardson MS, Cramer JT, Bemben DA, et al. Effects of age and ACL reconstruction on quadriceps gamma loop function. J Geriatr Phys Ther 2006;29(1):28–34.

[68] Konishi Y, Konishi H, Fukubayashi T. Gamma loop dysfunction in quadriceps on the contralateral side in patients with ruptured ACL. Med Sci Sports Exerc 2003;35(6):897–900.

[69] McNair PJ, Wood GA. Frequency analysis of the EMG from the quadriceps of the anterior cruciate ligament deficient individuals. Electromyogr Clin Neurophysiol 1993;33(1):43–8.

[70] Tsepis E, Vagenas G, Ristanis S, et al. Thigh muscle weakness in ACL-deficient knees persists without structured rehabilitation. Clin Orthop Relat Res 2006;450:211–8.

[71] St Clair Gibson A, Lambert MI, Durandt JJ, et al. Quadriceps and hamstrings peak torque ratio changes in persons with chronic anterior cruciate ligament deficiency. J Orthop Sports Phys Ther 2000;30(7):418–27.

[72] Lorentzon R, Elmqvist LG, Sjostrom M, et al. Thigh musculature in relation to chronic anterior cruciate ligament tear: muscle size, morphology, and mechanical output before reconstruction. Am J Sports Med 1989;17(3):423–9.

[73] Tsepis E, Vagenas G, Giakas G, et al. Hamstring weakness as an indicator of poor knee function in ACL-deficient patients. Knee Surg Sports Traumatol Arthrosc 2004;12(1):22–9.

[74] Hiemstra LA, Webber S, MacDonald PB, et al. Knee strength deficits after hamstring tendon and patellar tendon anterior cruciate ligament reconstruction. Med Sci Sports Exerc 2000;32(8):1472–9.

[75] Eastlack ME, Axe MJ, Snyder-Mackler L. Laxity, instability, and functional outcome after ACL injury: copers versus noncopers. Med Sci Sports Exerc 1999;31(2):210–5.

[76] Acierno SP, D'Ambrosia C, Solomonow M, et al. Electromyography and biomechanics of a dynamic knee brace for anterior cruciate ligament deficiency. Orthopedics 1995;18(11):1101–7.

[77] Anderson JL, Lamb SE, Barker KL, et al. Changes in muscle torque following anterior cruciate ligament reconstruction: a comparison between hamstrings and patella tendon graft procedures on 45 patients. Acta Orthop Scand 2002;73(5):546–52.

[78] Bryant AL, Kelly J, Hohmann E. Neuromuscular adaptations and correlates of knee functionality following ACL reconstruction. J Orthop Res 2008;26(1):126–35.

[79] de Jong S, van Caspel D, van Haeff M, et al. Functional assessment and muscle strength before and after reconstruction of chronic anterior cruciate ligament lesions. Arthroscopy 2007;23(1):21–8.

[80] Grossman MG, ElAttrache NS, Shields CL, et al. Revision anterior cruciate ligament reconstruction: three- to nine-year follow-up. Arthroscopy 2005;21(4):418–23.

[81] Hiemstra LA, Webber S, MacDonald PB, et al. Contralateral limb strength deficits after anterior cruciate ligament reconstruction using a hamstring tendon graft. Clin Biomech (Bristol, Avon) 2007;22(5):543–50.

[82] Jarvela T, Kannus P, Latvala K, et al. Simple measurements in assessing muscle performance after an ACL reconstruction. Int J Sports Med 2002;23(3):196–201.

[83] Keays SL, Bullock-Saxton J, Keays AC, et al. Muscle strength and function before and after anterior cruciate ligament reconstruction using semitendinosus and gracilis. Knee 2001;8(3):229–34.

[84] Kobayashi A, Higuchi H, Terauchi M, et al. Muscle performance after anterior cruciate ligament reconstruction. Int Orthop 2004;28(1):48–51.

[85] Konishi Y, Ikeda K, Nishino A, et al. Relationship between quadriceps femoris muscle volume and muscle torque after anterior cruciate ligament repair. Scand J Med Sci Sports 2007;17(6):656–61.

[86] Lee S, Seong SC, Jo H, et al. Outcome of anterior cruciate ligament reconstruction using quadriceps tendon autograft. Arthroscopy 2004;20(8):795–802.

[87] Mattacola CG, Perrin DH, Gansneder BM, et al. Strength, functional outcome, and postural stability after anterior cruciate ligament reconstruction. J Athl Train 2002;37(3): 262–8.

[88] Moisala AS, Jarvela T, Kannus P, et al. Muscle strength evaluations after ACL reconstruction. Int J Sports Med 2007;28(10):868–72.

[89] Nakamura N, Horibe S, Sasaki S, et al. Evaluation of active knee flexion and hamstring strength after anterior cruciate ligament reconstruction using hamstring tendons. Arthroscopy 2002;18(6):598–602.

[90] Nyland J, Caborn DN, Rothbauer J, et al. Two-year outcomes following ACL reconstruction with allograft tibialis anterior tendons: a retrospective study. Knee Surg Sports Traumatol Arthrosc 2003;11(4):212–8.

[91] Østeràs H, Augestad L, Tøndel S. Isokinetic muscle strength after anterior cruciate ligament reconstruction. Scand J Med Sci Sports 1998;8:279–82.

[92] Segawa H, Omori G, Koga Y, et al. Rotational muscle strength of the limb after anterior cruciate ligament reconstruction using semitendinosus and gracilis tendon. Arthroscopy 2002;18(2):177–82.

[93] Seto JL, Orofino AS, Morrissey MC, et al. Assessment of quadriceps/hamstring strength, knee ligament stability, functional and sports activity levels five years after anterior cruciate ligament reconstruction. Am J Sports Med 1988;16(2):170–80.

[94] Elmqvist LG, Lorentzon R, Johansson C, et al. Knee extensor muscle function before and after reconstruction of anterior cruciate ligament tear. Scand J Rehabil Med 1989; 21(3):131–9.

[95] Ageberg E, Pettersson A, Friden T. 15-year follow-up of neuromuscular function in patients with unilateral nonreconstructed anterior cruciate ligament injury initially treated with rehabilitation and activity modification: a longitudinal prospective study. Am J Sports Med 2007;35(12):2109–17.

[96] Blyth MJ, Gosal HS, Peake WM, et al. Anterior cruciate ligament reconstruction in patients over the age of 50 years: 2- to 8-year follow-up. Knee Surg Sports Traumatol Arthrosc 2003;11(4):204–11.

[97] Makihara Y, Nishino A, Fukubayashi T, et al. Decrease of knee flexion torque in patients with ACL reconstruction: combined analysis of the architecture and function of the knee flexor muscles. Knee Surg Sports Traumatol Arthrosc 2006;14(4):310–7.

[98] Tow BP, Chang PC, Mitra AK, et al. Comparing 2-year outcomes of anterior cruciate ligament reconstruction using either patella-tendon or semitendinosus-tendon autografts: a non-randomised prospective study. J Orthop Surg (Hong Kong) 2005;13(2):139–46.

[99] Baugher WH, Warren RF, Marshall JL, et al. Quadriceps atrophy in the anterior cruciate insufficient knee. Am J Sports Med 1984;12(3):192–5.

[100] Arangio GA, Chen C, Kalady M, et al. Thigh muscle size and strength after anterior cruciate ligament reconstruction and rehabilitation. J Orthop Sports Phys Ther 1997;26(5):238–43.

[101] Stockmar C, Lill H, Trapp A, et al. Fibre type related changes in the metabolic profile and fibre diameter of human vastus medialis muscle after anterior cruciate ligament rupture. Acta Histochem 2006;108(5):335–42.

[102] Williams GN, Snyder-Mackler L, Barrance PJ, et al. Quadriceps femoris muscle morphology and function after ACL injury: a differential response in copers versus non-copers. J Biomech 2005;38(4):685–93.

[103] Nishino A, Sanada A, Kanehisa H, et al. Knee-flexion torque and morphology of the semitendinosus after ACL reconstruction. Med Sci Sports Exerc 2006;38(11): 1895–900.

[104] Burks RT, Crim J, Fink BP, et al. The effects of semitendinosus and gracilis harvest in anterior cruciate ligament reconstruction. Arthroscopy 2005;21(10):1177–85.

[105] Irie K, Tomatsu T. Atrophy of semitendinosus and gracilis and flexor mechanism function after hamstring tendon harvest for anterior cruciate ligament reconstruction. Orthopedics 2002;25(5):491–5.

[106] Gerber JP, Marcus RL, Dibble LE, et al. Effects of early progressive eccentric exercise on muscle structure after anterior cruciate ligament reconstruction. J Bone Joint Surg Am 2007;89(3):559–70.

[107] Holm L, Esmarck B, Mizuno M, et al. The effect of protein and carbohydrate supplementation on strength training outcome of rehabilitation in ACL patients. J Orthop Res 2006;24(11):2114–23.

[108] Currier DP, Ray JM, Nyland J, et al. Effects of electrical and electromagnetic stimulation after anterior cruciate ligament reconstruction. J Orthop Sports Phys Ther 1993;17(4): 177–84.

[109] Takarada Y, Takazawa H, Ishii N. Applications of vascular occlusion diminish disuse atrophy of knee extensor muscles. Med Sci Sports Exerc 2000;32(12):2035–9.

[110] Lysholm M, Ledin T, Odkvist LM, et al. Postural control—a comparison between patients with chronic anterior cruciate ligament insufficiency and healthy individuals. Scand J Med Sci Sports 1998;8(6):432–8.

[111] O'Connell M, George K, Stock D. Postural sway and balance testing: a comparison of normal and anterior cruciate ligament deficient knees. Gait Posture 1998;8(2):136–42.

[112] Tecco S, Salini V, Calvisi V, et al. Effects of anterior cruciate ligament (ACL) injury on postural control and muscle activity of head, neck and trunk muscles. J Oral Rehabil 2006;33(8):576–87.

[113] Hoffman M, Schrader J, Koceja D. An investigation of postural control in postoperative anterior cruciate ligament reconstruction patients. J Athl Train 1999;34(2):130–6.

[114] Henriksson M, Ledin T, Good L. Postural control after anterior cruciate ligament reconstruction and functional rehabilitation. Am J Sports Med 2001;29(3):359–66.

[115] Rudolph KS, Eastlack ME, Axe MJ, et al. Movement patterns after anterior cruciate ligament injury: a comparison of patients who compensate well for the injury and those who require operative stabilization. J Electromyogr Kinesiol 1998;8(6):349–62.

[116] Snyder-Mackler L, Fitzgerald GK, Bartolozzi AR III, et al. The relationship between passive joint laxity and functional outcome after anterior cruciate ligament injury. Am J Sports Med 1997;25(2):191–5.

[117] Rudolph KS, Axe MJ, Buchanan TS, et al. Dynamic stability in the anterior cruciate ligament deficient knee. Knee Surg Sports Traumatol Arthrosc 2001;9(2):62–71.

[118] Knoll Z, Kiss RM, Kocsis L. Gait adaptation in ACL deficient patients before and after anterior cruciate ligament reconstruction surgery. J Electromyogr Kinesiol 2004;14(3): 287–94.

[119] Knoll Z, Kocsis L, Kiss R. Gait patterns before and after anterior cruciate ligament reconstruction. Knee Surg Sports Traumatol Arthrosc 2004;12(1):7–14.

[120] Berchuck M, Andriacchi TP, Bach BR, et al. Gait adaptations by patients who have a deficient anterior cruciate ligament. J Bone Joint Surg Am 1990;72(6):871–7.

[121] Alkjaer T, Simonsen EB, Jorgensen U, et al. Evaluation of the walking pattern in two types of patients with anterior cruciate ligament deficiency: copers and non-copers. Eur J Appl Physiol 2003;89(3–4):301–8.

[122] Hurd WJ, Snyder-Mackler L. Knee instability after acute ACL rupture affects movement patterns during the mid-stance phase of gait. J Orthop Res 2007;25(10):1369–77.

[123] Patel RR, Hurwitz DE, Andriacchi TP, et al. Mechanisms for the "quadriceps avoidance gait" seen in ACL deficient patients. Gait Posture 1997;5(2):147.

[124] Roberts CS, Rash GS, Honaker JT, et al. A deficient anterior cruciate ligament does not lead to quadriceps avoidance gait. Gait Posture 1999;10(3):189–99.

[125] Elias JJ, Faust AF, Chu YH, et al. The soleus muscle acts as an agonist for the anterior cruciate ligament. An in vitro experimental study. Am J Sports Med 2003;31(2):241–6.

[126] Devita P, Hortobagyi T, Barrier J, et al. Gait adaptations before and after anterior cruciate ligament reconstruction surgery. Med Sci Sports Exerc 1997;29:853–9.

[127] Ernst GP, Saliba E, Diduch DR, et al. Lower-extremity compensations following anterior cruciate ligament reconstruction. Phys Ther 2000;80(3):251–60.

[128] Irrgang JJ, Ho H, Harner CD, et al. Use of the International Knee Documentation Committee guidelines to assess outcome following anterior cruciate ligament reconstruction. Knee Surg Sports Traumatol Arthrosc 1998;6(2):107–14.

[129] Irrgang JJ, Anderson AF, Boland AL, et al. Development and validation of the international knee documentation committee subjective knee form. Am J Sports Med 2001;29(5):600–13.

[130] Irrgang JJ, Anderson AF, Boland AL, et al. Responsiveness of the International Knee Documentation Committee Subjective Knee Form. Am J Sports Med 2006;34(10):1567–73.

[131] Anderson AF, Irrgang JJ, Kocher MS, et al. The International Knee Documentation Committee Subjective Knee Evaluation Form: normative data. Am J Sports Med 2006;34(1):128–35.

[132] Tegner Y, Lysholm J. Rating systems in the evaluation of knee ligament injuries. Clin Orthop Relat Res Sep 1985;198:43–9.

[133] Flandry F, Hunt JP, Terry GC, et al. Analysis of subjective knee complaints using visual analog scales. Am J Sports Med 1991;19(2):112–8.

[134] Barber-Westin SD, Noyes FR, McCloskey JW. Rigorous statistical reliability, validity, and responsiveness testing of the Cincinnati knee rating system in 350 subjects with uninjured, injured, or anterior cruciate ligament-reconstructed knees. Am J Sports Med 1999;27(4):402–16.

[135] Bellamy N, Buchanan WW, Goldsmith CH, et al. Validation study of WOMAC: a health status instrument for measuring clinically important patient relevant outcomes to antirheumatic drug therapy in patients with osteoarthritis of the hip or knee. J Rheumatol 1988;15(12):1833–40.

[136] Roos EM, Roos HP, Lohmander LS, et al. Knee Injury and Osteoarthritis Outcome Score (KOOS)–development of a self-administered outcome measure. J Orthop Sports Phys Ther 1998;28(2):88–96.

[137] Pinczewski LA, Lyman J, Salmon LJ, et al. A 10-year comparison of anterior cruciate ligament reconstructions with hamstring tendon and patellar tendon autograft: a controlled, prospective trial. Am J Sports Med 2007;35(4):564–74.

[138] Laxdal G, Kartus J, Hansson L, et al. A prospective randomized comparison of bone-patellar tendon-bone and hamstring grafts for anterior cruciate ligament reconstruction. Arthroscopy 2005;21(1):34–42.

[139] Laxdal G, Sernert N, Ejerhed L, et al. A prospective comparison of bone-patellar tendon-bone and hamstring tendon grafts for anterior cruciate ligament reconstruction in male patients. Knee Surg Sports Traumatol Arthrosc Sep 9 2007;15(2):115–25.
[140] Hurd WJ, Axe MJ, Snyder-Mackler L. A 10-year prospective trial of a patient management algorithm and screening examination for highly active individuals with anterior cruciate ligament injury: part 1, outcomes. Am J Sports Med 2008;36(1):40–7.
[141] Quinby JS, Golish SR, Hart JA, et al. All-inside meniscal repair using a new flexible, tensionable device. Am J Sports Med Feb 21 2006;34(8):1281–6.
[142] Nebelung W, Wuschech H. Thirty-five years of follow-up of anterior cruciate ligament-deficient knees in high-level athletes. Arthroscopy 2005;21(6):696–702.
[143] Salmon LJ, Refshauge KM, Russell VJ, et al. Gender differences in outcome after anterior cruciate ligament reconstruction with hamstring tendon autograft. Am J Sports Med 2006;34(4):621–9.
[144] Ferrari JD, Bach BR Jr, Bush-Joseph CA, et al. Anterior cruciate ligament reconstruction in men and women: An outcome analysis comparing gender. Arthroscopy 2001;17(6):588–96.
[145] Carter TR, Edinger S. Isokinetic evaluation of anterior ligament reconstruction: hamstring versus patellar tendon. Arthroscopy 1999;15(2):169–72.

Clin Sports Med 27 (2008) 405–424

CLINICS IN SPORTS MEDICINE

Maximizing Quadriceps Strength After ACL Reconstruction

Riann M. Palmieri-Smith, PhD, ATC[a,b,c,*],
Abbey C. Thomas, MEd, ATC[a], Edward M. Wojtys, MD[b,c]

[a]Division of Kinesiology, University of Michigan, 401 Washtenaw Avenue,
Ann Arbor, MI 48109-2214, USA
[b]Department of Orthopaedic Surgery, University of Michigan, 1500 East Medical Center Drive,
2912 Taubman Center, Box 0328, Ann Arbor, MI 48109, USA
[c]Bone and Joint Injury Prevention and Rehabilitation Center, University of Michigan, Domino
Farms, 24 Frank Lloyd Wright Drive, MedSport, Lobby A, Ann Arbor, MI 48106, USA

The primary objectives of anterior cruciate ligament (ACL) surgery and rehabilitation are to restore knee function to preinjury levels and promote long-
term joint health. Despite the best efforts of physicians and rehabilitation
professionals, often these goals are not achieved, as many patients return to sport
with lingering neuromuscular deficits and often are plagued with symptoms associated with the premature development of osteoarthritis. Quadriceps weakness is
among the persistent neuromuscular deficiencies associated with ACL injury [1–
3] and presents a major rehabilitation challenge for patients and clinicians alike [4].

Rehabilitation of the quadriceps musculature following ACL reconstruction often has been the subject of much debate. In fact, in the late 1970s and early 1980s,
strengthening of the quadriceps was downplayed because of concerns that exercise
may place excessive strain on the ACL graft, while today, early, aggressive
strengthening of this muscle group is advocated, as evidence has mounted that
most quadriceps exercises are safe [5] and necessary to maximize knee joint function [6–17]. Although clinicians and scientists continue to make strides toward improving current rehabilitation techniques and developing new interventions to
maximize quadriceps output following ACL reconstruction, a universally effective
means by which to restore preinjury muscle strength still has not been uncovered.
Thus, even when surgical intervention and rehabilitation are deemed successful
and patients return to sport, full quadriceps strength often has not been achieved.

An examination of the current literature suggests that quadriceps strength
deficits can exceed 20% at 6 months post-ACL reconstruction, a time when
many athletes are cleared to return to activity (Table 1) [18–56]. The magnitude of quadriceps weakness appears to lessen with time, but most research

*Corresponding author. Division of Kinesiology, University of Michigan, 4745G CCRB,
401 Washtenaw Avenue, Ann Arbor, MI 48109-2214. E-mail address: riannp@umich.edu
(R.M. Palmieri-Smith).

0278-5919/08/$ – see front matter
doi:10.1016/j.csm.2008.02.001

Table 1
Summary of studies evaluating isokinetic knee extension strength measured at 60°/seconds in anterior cruciate ligament reconstructed patients

Author	N	Time after reconstruction (months)	Graft type	Quadriceps deficit (%)
Anderson [18]	70	$\bar{x} = 84$	SG	7
Anderson [19]	35	$\bar{x} = 35.4$	PT	14
	33		SG	4
Anderson JL [19]	22	6	PT	28.7
	23		ST	21.3
		12	PT	18.7
			ST	20.5
Aune [20]	35	6	PT	25
	37		SG	12
		12	PT	10
			SG	10
		24	PT	10
			SG	10
Beard [21]	26	3	PT	39
		6		29
Beynnon [22]	28	12	PT	16.5
	28		ST	15.2
		36	PT	5.3
			ST	11.9
Boden [23]	20	$\bar{x} = 26$	SG	9
Cardone [24]	67	4	PT	33
		6		25
Chen [25]	62	$\bar{x} = 28$	SG	6.5
Feller [26]	28	4	PT	36.3
	34		ST	27.2
	24	8	PT	25.5
	33		ST	12.1
	21	12	PT	22.7
	18		ST	11.1
Giron [27]	43	5	SG	37.5
		12		5
		24		3.5
		60		3.3
Gobbi [28]	40	3	PT	40
	40		ST	31
		5	PT	31.5
			ST	22
		12	PT	12.5
			ST	12.5
Gobbi [29]	80	3	ST	22.8
		6		15.6
		12		7.5
Gokeler [30]	14	6	PT	25.1
Goradia [31]	85	$\bar{x} = 44$	SG	<10
Hamada [32]	106	24	ST	10.8
Hofmeister [33]	17	$\bar{x} = 31$	Mixed	20.1
Jansson [34]	99	12	PT	21
			ST	15
Jarvela [35]	86	$\bar{x} = 84$	PT	10.3
Keays [36]	31	6	PT	28.6
Keays [37]	31	6	SG	12

(continued on next page)

Table 1
(continued)

Author	N	Time after reconstruction (months)	Graft type	Quadriceps deficit (%)
Keays [8]	31	6	SG	7.3
Keays [38]	29	72	PT	6
	27		ST	−1.7
Kobayashi [39]	36	1	PT	66.9
		6		36.8
		12		27.1
		24		10.9
Larkin [40]	34	$\bar{x} = 30.5$	PT	5.5
Lee [41]	67	6	PT	28
		12		18
		24		18
Lephart [42]	15	$\bar{x} = 18.6$	PT	5
Maeda [43]	41	$\bar{x} = 27$	Mixed	10.3
Marder [44]	37	$\bar{x} = 29$	PT	12
	35		SG	9
McHugh [45]	102	6	Mixed	33
Moisala [46]	16	72	PT	10
	28		SG	7
Natri [47]	119	46.8	PT	17.5
Osteras [48]	90	$\bar{x} = 6.75$	PT	28.7
Petersen [49]	27[a]	$\bar{x} = 4.3$	PT	16.7
	37[b]			13.7
Pokar [50]	76	$\bar{x} = 60$	PT	2.1
Reat [51]	27	$\bar{x} = 16$	PT	25
Rosenberg [52]	10	$\bar{x} = 17.9$	PT	18
Segawa [53]	62	12	Mixed	7.1
Soon [54]	76	3	SG	33.9
		6		8.2
Tashiro [55]	49	6	ST	25
	36		SG	28
		12	ST	17
			SG	20
		18	ST	8
			SG	10
Witvrouw [56]	17	6	PT	40.5
	32		SG	37.6
		12	PT	23.2
			SG	16.5
Wojtys [16]	25	6	PT	24
		12		14
		18		10

Negative values indicate injured leg is stronger than uninjured leg.

Abbreviations: PT, patellar tendon; ST, semitendinosus; SG, semitendinosus + gracilis.

[a]Indicates acute injury before reconstruction (time to reconstruction = 1–21 days).

[b]Indicates chronic injury before reconstruction (time to reconstruction = 10–12 weeks).

suggests that deficits are apparent between the injured and uninjured limb years following reconstruction, illustrating the long-term nature of this problem. Also of concern, is the mounting evidence suggesting that bilateral quadriceps weakness is present following unilateral ACL injury [57–59]. As the quadriceps is critical to dynamic joint stability, and weakness of this muscle group is related to poor functional outcomes [6–10,12–14,16,17,60] and may contribute to the early onset of osteoarthritis [61], identifying strategies to minimize quadriceps weakness following ACL injury and reconstruction is of great clinical interest. Therefore, the purpose of this article is to review the current literature and critically discuss current rehabilitation approaches to restore quadriceps muscle function after ACL reconstruction.

ETIOLOGY OF QUADRICEPS WEAKNESS: SHOULD THIS INFLUENCE REHABILITATION STRATEGY?

Before initiating ACL rehabilitation programs, clinicians often set a goal of improving/maximizing their patients' quadriceps strength. Although this goal is appropriate and worthwhile, the ability to achieve it is directly dependent on the factors that are responsible for the resultant muscle weakness. A failure to completely understand the potential underlying contributors to the quadriceps weakness likely will result in the development of ineffective rehabilitation strategies and ultimately failure to achieve this goal. Although a definite etiology for the quadriceps weakness associated with ACL injury and reconstruction remains elusive, there is evidence to suggest that arthrogenic muscle inhibition (AMI) and perhaps muscle atrophy are primarily responsible for the decrements in quadriceps strength.

Arthrogenic muscle inhibition (eg, voluntary activation failure) is hypothesized to result from reflex activity in which altered afference originating from the injured joint leads to a diminished efferent motor drive to the muscles [62]. Specifically, loss of mechanoreceptors from the ACL is thought to disrupt the ligamentous–muscular reflex between the ACL and the quadriceps, leading to an inability to actively recruit high-threshold motor units during voluntary quadriceps contractions. AMI has been identified almost universally in all studies examining quadriceps activation in patients after ACL rupture and reconstruction (Table 2). Maybe more importantly, it has been shown to contribute to the ever-present post-traumatic quadriceps strength deficits [1,3,58,59,63–65]. It is also important to note that AMI presents bilaterally following unilateral ACL rupture and surprisingly, in some cases, the quadriceps activation failure in the contralateral limb is reported to be equivalent to that of the injured limb [66].[1]

---

[1]Bilateral activation deficits call into question the use of the quadriceps index as a measure of quadriceps strength. The quadriceps index, computed by dividing the peak torque of the injured limb by the peak torque of the uninjured limb and multiplying that value by 100, treats the uninjured leg as the control leg and is assumed to represent a subject's normal, preinjury quadriceps strength. As bilateral activation deficits appear to be present, it is likely that the quadriceps index underestimates true muscle strength deficits. Thus, if choosing to use this measure to assess strength, an adjustment for activation must be considered. Because no adjustments were made in any of the studies presented in Table 1, it can be assumed that the quadriceps strength deficits would be higher than what is reported by the authors.

Table 2
Summary of studies evaluating quadriceps activation deficits in anterior cruciate ligament-deficient and reconstructed limbs

Author	N	Time since injury (months)	Measurement technique	Quadriceps activation deficit (%)
Chmielewski [63]	100	$\bar{x} = 1.5$	Burst superimposition	7.4 (I)
				7.2 (U)
Snyder-Mackler [64]	20[a]	$\bar{x} = 2$[b]	Burst superimposition	25[c]
	12	$\bar{x} = 3$[b]		21[c]
	8	$\bar{x} = 24$		25[c]
Urbach [59]	22	Median $= 3.9$	Interpolated twitch	21 (I)
				20 (U)
Urbach [3]	12[d]	24[b]	Interpolated twitch	14.7 (I)
				16 (U)

Abbreviations: I, involved; U, uninvolved.
[a]Indicates Achilles tendon allograft and semitendinosus autograft used in reconstruction.
[b]Indicates time since reconstruction.
[c]Value reported as percent deficits between limbs.
[d]Indicates semitendinosus autograft reconstruction.

A diminished ability to voluntarily activate the quadriceps (eg, AMI) may provide an explanation for the lingering quadriceps weakness following ACL rupture and subsequent repair and rehabilitation. Often the strengthening components of ACL rehabilitation are focused on exercises that require patients to voluntarily activate their muscles. As AMI prevents complete voluntary activation, typical rehabilitation protocols focused on active 'exercise, but are likely to be ineffective and will limit the ability to achieve the patients' complete recovery of strength. Furthermore, because quadriceps activation failure is present bilaterally after ACL injury and surgery, rehabilitation protocols focused on the injured limb only are not comprehensive and likely will result in persistent neuromuscular deficits.

Quadriceps muscle atrophy, a decrease in the size of the skeletal muscle, often is apparent following ACL rupture and reconstruction, but its origin is unknown, and its contribution to quadriceps weakness remains debatable. Most research has established little relationship between muscle atrophy and the magnitude of quadriceps weakness associated with ACL injury [67,68]. Contrary to these findings, Williams and colleagues [69] recently showed that quadriceps atrophy and activation failure together account for approximately 62% of the variance in the quadriceps weakness of ACL-deficient noncopers, suggesting atrophy plays a significant role in reducing quadriceps strength. Whether atrophy persists following ACL reconstruction and rehabilitation and contributes to long-term quadriceps weakness has not been examined and requires future study.

As atrophy likely plays some role in post-traumatic quadriceps weakness, one must consider its origin to effectively employ appropriate treatment. Typically, the disuse atrophy that occurs with ACL injury is considered to result from decreased exercise intensity/volume from the lack of participation in sport and/or immobilization of the knee joint. In this case, using voluntary exercise to aid in the restoration of muscle hypertrophy appears warranted. One must consider, however, that the quadriceps atrophy associated with ACL injury is likely, at least in part, caused by the presence AMI. Remember, AMI prevents complete activation of the quadriceps and therefore can generate a body-induced disuse, whereby the lack of tension produced in the inhibited muscle fibers leads to atrophy of the affected tissue. Thus, if one could prevent AMI, one likely would be able to reduce the magnitude of quadriceps atrophy.

In summary, the source of quadriceps muscle weakness must be considered when designing rehabilitation protocols. Using one strategy (eg, voluntary exercise) to regain complete quadriceps strength likely will result in incomplete muscle recovery and should be avoided.

METHODS TO MAXIMIZE QUADRICEPS STRENGTH

The focus of this section is to provide some insight regarding potential therapeutic interventions that may aid the clinician in maximizing muscle strength. There are numerous strategies that may be effective for minimizing AMI and muscle atrophy. Therefore, rehabilitation methods will be discussed in two major major sections: approaches to minimize AMI and approaches to minimize muscle atrophy.

Therapeutic Approaches to Minimizing Arthrogenic Muscle Inhibition

Most clinicians do not incorporate a goal of minimizing muscle inhibition in their current ACL rehabilitation programs. Rather, most programs are developed around minimizing atrophy and recovering full muscle strength. It often is not considered that if one fails to overcome muscle inhibition one will be unable to achieve goals to retard atrophy and regain full strength. Thus, the authors strongly contend that clinicians shift their efforts to preventing/removing AMI. If clinicians are effective in combating AMI early in the rehabilitation process, they will minimize the resulting strength deficits and diminish the muscle atrophy, which should lead to a more complete and more effective program and likely will result in quicker patient recovery and return to sport.

So the question becomes, how can one target muscle inhibition? To remove AMI, one needs to alter the inhibitory processes resulting in it by using one of two strategies: altering afferent feedback that signals something is wrong with the knee, or modifying the motor drive at the motor axon or from the motor cortex that ultimately leads to the muscle shutdown. Rehabilitation approaches to target AMI are discussed in two sections; each part will focus on one side of the problem (the sensory side and the motor side).

Removing arthrogenic muscle inhibition: targeting the sensory side of the problem
AMI can be caused by increased afferent activity, evidenced by joint effusion, or by a lack of afferent activity, which may be the case with a loss of mechanoreceptors subsequent to an ACL rupture. Thus, one approach to preventing AMI would be blocking/modifying the sensory signals responsible for initiating

the inhibitory process. This might be achieved by removing abnormal afferent stimuli, minimizing pain, or sending signals to the central nervous system that may modify presynaptic pathways contributing to AMI.

Minimizing joint effusion. Minimizing joint effusion is a very important goal associated with the rehabilitation of ACL reconstructed patients. Clinicians recognize that reducing the effusion will result in increased range of motion and decreased pain, and will improve overall joint function. Although often not considered, minimizing a knee effusion likely will reduce the amount of AMI.

Aspiration of a knee joint effusion has been shown to increase integrated electromyogram (EMG) in patients with chronic knee effusions [70]. Further, removal of an artificially induced joint effusion leads to improvements in quadriceps strength [71]. Aspirating postoperative knee effusions that do not resolve after few days is a good way to reduce the magnitude of quadriceps inhibition. Although there are some risks associated with aspiration, these can be minimized by using excellent sterile technique. If clinicians are not comfortable aspirating fluid from the knee, the authors strongly encourage the use of any therapeutic means necessary to minimize fluid within the capsule as soon as possible (eg, compression, electrical stimulation, and elevation). Removing the effusion, which contributes to abnormal afference, will aid in minimizing AMI and maximizing quadriceps output.

Cryotherapy. Cryotherapy often is applied early in ACL rehabilitation to retard inflammation and reduce pain, but cooling of the knee joint also may serve to decrease AMI. Cold is capable of decreasing nerve conduction velocity [72,73] and slowing the discharge rate of joint mechanoreceptors [74], which could result in diminished afferents being delivered to the central nervous system and possibly a decrease in inhibition. Another rationale for why cold may be an effective therapy to remove AMI would be its ability to diminish pain. It should be noted, however, that although pain is often considered to cause AMI, this theory is not always supported by existing literature [75–77].

Hopkins and colleagues [78] found that application of ice to the knee joint for 30 minutes was capable of completely reversing AMI of the vastus medialis that resulted from an induced knee joint effusion. Surprisingly, they also noted that the cryotherapy treatment resulted in a facilitation of the quadriceps (eg, after the ice treatment the motoneuron excitability was higher than it was before the effusion) (Fig. 1). The facilitation of the muscle suggests that ice might not only reverse inhibition by modifying afferent feedback, but that it may affect central commands also [78]. In this study, the effects of the cryotherapy treatment lasted after the ice was removed and remained for at least 60 minutes (measurements ceased at 60 minutes, and the muscle was still facilitated). In a follow-up study, Hopkins [79] noted that cryotherapy was capable of negating movement deficiencies associated with an effusion induced inhibition. Together, these results suggest that cold application to the knee joint is not only capable of removing quadriceps inhibition, but can minimize its associated functional deficits. Although the previously mentioned results are promising and suggest that

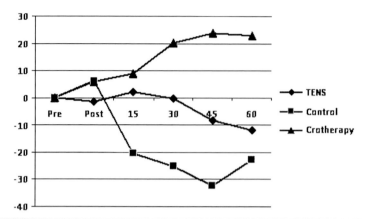

Fig. 1. H-reflex amplitudes over time expressed as percentage change from the preinjection measurement. Measures were recorded before and following injection of saline into the knee joint capsule and then either cryotherapy, Transcutaneous electrical nerve stimulation (TENS), or no treatment were applied, and H-reflex measurements were gathered at 15, 30, and 60 minutes. At 30 minutes, the cryotherapy or TENS treatment was removed, and then the H-reflex was recorded. Values greater than 0 indicate quadriceps facilitation, while values less than 0 represent quadriceps inhibition. (*Adapted from* Hopkins JT, Ingersoll CD, Edwards JE, et al. Cryotherapy and transcutaneous electric neuromuscular stimulation decrease arthrogenic muscle inhibition of the vastus medialis after knee joint effusion. J Athl Train 2002;37: 25–31; with permission.)

cryotherapy may be an effective way to temporarily reverse AMI, they must be put into context. The effects of cryotherapy on quadriceps inhibition, in the previously mentioned studies, were examined using an effusion model. The effusion model elicits inhibition in the absence of true injury, inflammation, and pain, and the results cannot be assumed to apply to actual injury. At this time, there is no information as to whether cryotherapy is an effective means of reversing AMI in the ACL patient. Despite this fact, the authors would encourage clinicians to apply ice before engaging patients in early active exercise (eg, quad sets and straight leg raises) following ACL reconstruction because of its potential to maximize quadriceps muscle function.

Transcutaneous electrical nerve stimulation. Transcutaneous electrical nerve stimulation (TENS) sometimes is used in ACL rehabilitation in an attempt to combat pain, but like cryotherapy, it also may be an effective intervention to reduce AMI. Stimulation of cutaneous nerves, the nerves excited during TENS treatments, has been shown to reduce presynaptic inhibition [80], and as presynaptic inhibition appears to contribute to mediating AMI [81], TENS may be an appropriate therapy to use in ACL rehabilitation. TENS also may act to reverse AMI by altering afferent signals that result in a reduction of joint pain.

Hopkins and colleagues [78], in the same study where they evaluated the effects of cryotherapy on AMI, tried to determine if TENS could reverse the quadriceps inhibition in people who have an induced knee effusion. During the 30-minute TENS treatment, the quadriceps was disinhibited (eg, the quadriceps excitability returned to baseline levels), but when the stimulator was turned off, the inhibition gradually returned (see Fig. 1). TENS also has led to small increases in maximum quadriceps contractions in patients after ACL reconstruction [82] and open mensicectomy [77], but the noted effects were small and likely would not improve clinical outcome. The application of TENS in these latter two studies must be considered, however. Both of the studies done postsurgically assessed quadriceps strength after the TENS unit had been turned off. It would appear, based on the findings of Hopkins and colleagues [78], that TENS provides the greatest advantage while the unit is turned on, and clinicians wishing to use this intervention to reverse AMI should use it in this way. In clinical practice, the authors use TENS as it was studied by Arvidsson and Eriksson [82] and Stokes and colleagues [77], with a patient sitting on a table while receiving some other type of therapy, often an ice bag. The authors would suggest that TENS should be applied while patients are performing active exercise to maximize its potential to reduce AMI. Remember, AMI is a reduced ability to recruit motoneurons controlling the quadriceps muscle. If, while TENS is on, it diminishes inhibition and allows recruitment of otherwise unrecruitable motoneurons, then performing exercises during this time will allow clinicians to activate more of the muscle and hopefully diminish AMI and its negative consequences.

Anesthetics. Local anesthetics also may reverse AMI. Similar to cryotherapy and TENS, anesthetics may reduce AMI by means of the reduction of pain. It is just as plausible, however, that they may reduce AMI by blocking other afferents contributing to the inhibition. Keep in mind, AMI persists once pain has subsided and can be induced in the absence of pain (eg, the effusion model does not cause pain [78] but results in AMI); therefore rehabilitation strategies effective in removing AMI should not be focused solely on removing painful stimuli.

Injection of lidocaine into the knee joint capsule has been shown to improve isometric muscle strength in osteoarthritis patients [83]. Arvidsson and colleagues [84] noted increased integrated EMG activity in patients after ACL reconstruction following administration of a Lidocaine epidural. These results suggest that anesthetics may improve quadriceps activation associated with knee joint injury or disease. Practical methods for delivering these agents, however, are needed that minimize or eliminate the risks and/or adverse effects. Another consideration is that total blockade of pain is not desirable, as pain serves as a guide for patients and clinicians, indicating if the selected treatments and/or exercise regimens are appropriate at the current stage of healing. So, although local anesthetics maybe useful, one must consider their appropriateness in ACL rehabilitation. The authors first would employ other, more practical interventions mentioned in this article to remove AMI in the ACL reconstructed patient.

Topical anesthetics, in the form of sprays or ointments, might be a better alternative to local anesthetics; however, their effectiveness in reversing AMI has not been evaluated. A topical anesthetic sprayed over the soleus muscle and delivered by means of iontophoresis in healthy people was capable of increasing motoneuron activation, as measured by the H-reflex, suggesting that cutaneous afferents may be able to aid in minimizing muscle inhibition [85,86].

Removing arthrogenic muscle inhibition: targeting the motor side of the problem
Rather than blocking or modifying afferent traffic, an alternative approach to targeting AMI is to activate the inhibited motoneurons directly or to modify inhibitory signals from the brain that ultimately result in the muscle shutdown.

Neuromuscular electrical stimulation. Neuromuscular electrical stimulation (NMES) appears to be a promising intervention to use after ACL injury and reconstruction, when the clinician's rehabilitation goal is targeting AMI. As AMI prevents the active recruitment of quadriceps motoneurons, and electrical stimulation allows for the direct activation of the motor axon, NMES could allow for the direct recruitment of the inhibited motoneurons. Furthermore, muscle activation by means of NMES allows for the recruitment of a greater proportion of type 2 muscle fibers when compared with voluntary contractions of a similar intensity [87–89]. As type 2 muscle fibers are essential to achieve a higher level of quadriceps force production, their recruitment by means of NMES undoubtedly will aid in the quest to achieve complete recovery of quadriceps strength.

The existing literature predominately supports that NMES combined with active exercise is more effective than active exercise alone in restoring quadriceps strength following ACL reconstruction [90–95]. Snyder-Mackler and colleagues [65,93,94] demonstrated that 4 weeks of active exercise combined with high-intensity electrical stimulation resulted in quadriceps strength of about 70.1% of the uninjured leg at 2 months postreconstruction, while patients who received active exercise only had quadriceps strength of 46.7% of the uninjured limb. Similarly, Delitto and colleagues [90] reported that patients receiving NMES therapy had isometric strength of 78.8%, and those in an active exercise group only produced 51.7% at 8 weeks after ACL reconstruction.

The strength gains achieved by NMES appear to translate into an improvement in functional outcomes. Snyder-Mackler and colleagues [94] noted that patients who had received NMES walked with a faster cadence and velocity and spent more time during the stance phase on their involved limb. Furthermore, the NMES group displayed a more normal knee flexion excursion compared with those patients receiving active exercise. Overall, these results suggest that the quadriceps-induced strength gains, achieved through NMES, translate to functional improvements.

One of the downfalls of NMES is that some patients are not able to tolerate the prescribed protocols. The most effective procedures consist of subjects sitting in a dynamometer with the knee positioned in 60° to 95° of knee flexion and the stimulus applied at an intensity that induces at least 50% of a maximum voluntary isometric contraction. The high intensity of the stimulus and the knee flexion angles at which the tests are performed can be too uncomfortable for some patients. To accommodate for these issues, Fitzgerald and colleagues

[92] adapted the effective NMES protocols used by Snyder-Mackler [65,93,94] and Delitto and colleagues [90] in order to make the therapy more comfortable for patients. In their trial, NMES was delivered when the knee was in full extension, and the stimulus was applied so that it resulted in a full tetanic contraction and then was increased to maximum patient tolerance. The authors found that patients in the NMES plus exercise group demonstrated greater quadriceps strength and reported better functional status compared with the active exercise only group; however the strength gains noted were not as large in magnitude as those reported in previous works. Their results suggest that incorporating the modified NMES protocol into standard ACL rehabilitation is warranted when the ideal NMES paradigm is not tolerated by patients.

At this point, there are still some unanswered questions in regards to the effectiveness of NMES therapy. The primary question is how long do the strength gains achieved by NMES remain. The available research in ACL reconstructed patients provides evidence of the therapy's short-term effectiveness (eg, the early postoperative period, the first 4 to 8 weeks), but no data exist to suggest how long the strength gains remain after the NMES therapy ceases. Stevens and colleagues [96] noted that quadriceps activation was improved in patients following total knee arthroplasty after a 6-week NMES plus exercise program and that activation remained improved for up to 6 months following completion of treatment. Similar work is needed to determine if a lasting effect occurs in the treatment of ACL patients. If NMES is to provide maximum benefit in ACL rehabilitation, its results must prove to be sustained.

In summary, the incorporation of NMES therapy into ACL rehabilitation appears warranted. This intervention has been successful more than voluntary exercise alone in restoring quadriceps strength. Further, these gains in strength translate into improved functional outcomes.

Biofeedback. Biofeedback is a therapeutic technique whereby sensory or motor stimuli are provided to patients performing voluntary muscle contraction in an attempt to improve voluntary muscle control. This therapy is used to aid patients in developing a greater awareness of, and an increase in, voluntary control over their physiologic processes (eg, motor unit recruitment) that are otherwise involuntary and unfelt [97]. EMG is the most common signal used to provide feedback in knee rehabilitation [98–101], but temperature, verbal, pressure, and positional feedback also have proven successful in helping various patients regain muscle function [97,102,103].

Biofeedback therapy might be useful in overcoming muscle inhibition, although its efficacy in reversing AMI has yet to be proven. The mechanisms by which biofeedback may work remain unknown, but it has been suggested that this therapy may be able to alter the control of descending motor pathways [104]. Basmajian [104] has demonstrated with the use of visual and auditory signals that patients can control the recruitment of and the discharge frequency of motor units, which could lead to greater development of muscle tension. Simply put, the use of biofeedback in ACL rehabilitation may aid patients in overriding the inhibitory commands from the brain/spinal cord that ultimately have prevented activation of the affected motoneurons (eg, AMI). This ability to override inhibitory signals may allow patients to selectively recruit the otherwise unrecruitable motoneurons. Additionally, biofeedback may allow patients to more efficiently, through faster motor unit firing, recruit the already available motoneurons [104].

Maitland [105] found that EMG biofeedback, incorporated into a program of closed kinetic chain exercise, was able to reduce quadriceps AMI by 52% and increase knee extension peak torque by 203% in a single patient 8 months subsequent to ACL reconstruction who had reported progressively worsening knee instability. Further, it was shown that the increases in strength resulted in improved gait and decreased knee instability. In a study [101] examining the effectiveness of EMG biofeedback in patients who had undergone a meniscectomy, a 10-fold increase in quadriceps muscle activation was noted when compared with a standard rehabilitation group. Draper [98,99] noted that biofeedback along with standard rehabilitation was able to induce small increases in peak torque over a - week treatment period in postsurgical ACL patients.

Clinically speaking, the results presented suggest that EMG biofeedback could diminish quadriceps AMI and improve lower extremity function following ACL injury and reconstruction. More research must be done to prove its effectiveness and also to determine whether improvements in strength are caused by the removal of inhibition or occur because of a minimization of muscle atrophy.

Minimizing Muscle Atrophy

Typical ACL rehabilitation protocols already include techniques to combat muscle atrophy and recover strength in an uninhibited muscle. Active exercises are incorporated to regain strength, power, and endurance in the muscle surrounding the injured knee and will be increased in load and intensity as patients progress through the rehabilitation process. Although various resistance training programs have been introduced that allow for some recovery muscle strength and minimization of muscle atrophy, here only new and controversial approaches to reduce muscle atrophy are discussed in an attempt to aid clinicians in improving their current ACL rehabilitation programs.

Eccentric exercise (negative resistance training)

A muscle's force-producing capability is at its greatest when an external force surpasses that of the muscle and the muscle lengthens [106]. Thus, because the potential to overload the muscle is greater with negative training, increases in muscle size and strength should be of a larger magnitude when compared with standard concentric training. The use of progressive, high-intensity, lengthening (eccentric) contractions has been shown to be effective at improving muscle strength in young [107–109] and old [110] adults and patients with neurologic dysfunction [111,112]. Thus incorporating negative resistance training into postsurgical ACL rehabilitation presents an attractive option to aid in the restoration of muscle strength.

Preliminary evidence suggests that focused negative resistance training is successful in improving quadriceps muscle strength and in reducing quadriceps atrophy early after ACL reconstruction [113–115]. Gerber and colleagues [113] noted that patients who underwent a standard ACL rehabilitation protocol along with negative resistance training had a twofold greater increase in quadriceps peak cross-sectional area and volume compared with patients who received standard rehabilitation only. Further, quadriceps strength gains were greater in the patients who completed the negative training. The negative training employed in the previously mentioned study also diminished the atrophic changes in the uninvolved quadriceps.

Of clinical concern is the safety of performing such high-intensity lengthening muscle contractions, as forces of this type can induce muscle damage and also might be detrimental to the healing graft. Gerber's work [113] showed that progressive, gradual negative exercise is capable of inducing quadriceps hypertrophy without any apparent detrimental effects. Anterior knee laxity did not differ between the eccentric and standard rehabilitation groups, and the authors reported no cases of muscle damage as a result of the training.

Introducing focused negative exercise into ACL rehabilitation appears warranted to reduce disuse quadriceps atrophy. It should be noted that the long-term effects of negative training on quadriceps function are unknown and need to be studied further.

Open kinetic chain exercise versus closed kinetic chain exercise

The use of open kinetic chain (OKC) exercise in ACL rehabilitation has been the subject of much debate. OKC exercises have been shown to produce larger anterior shear forces than do closed kinetic chain (CKC) exercises and thus may be harmful to the healing graft. Because of their potential detrimental effects, the use of OKC exercises in postsurgical ACL rehabilitation has been questioned. On the other hand, the use of OKC exercises in ACL rehabilitation may be beneficial to the weakened quadriceps, as OKC exercise can task the affected muscle considerably. Thus, if OKC activities are found to be safe, incorporating these types of exercises might prove beneficial in minimizing muscle atrophy and improving strength after ACL reconstruction.

Unfortunately, examination of the current literature does not provide a definitive answer as to whether OKC exercises should be incorporated to ACL rehabilitation. Some studies have shown that OKC exercises or OKC plus CKC exercises are more effective than CKC exercises alone in improving quadriceps strength after ACL reconstruction [116,117] and in patients who are ACL deficient [118]. Others have found no differences in patients' quadriceps strength when comparing the two types of exercises [117,119]. Additionally, some research has shown that anterior knee laxity increases as a result of including OKC exercises in rehabilitation [116], while others have found no such difference [117,120].

In vivo measurements of ACL strain suggest that OKC exercises may not produce significantly more ACL strain that CKC. Beynnon and Fleming [121] have shown that peak ACL strains during OKC exercises were similar

Table 3
Summary of studies evaluating atrophy in ACL-deficient and reconstructed limbs

Author	N	Time since injury (months)	Measurement technique	Quadriceps CSA (cm^2)
Elmqvist [67]	11	median = 28	CT	64.9 (I)
				69.2 (U)
Lorentzon [68]	18	$\bar{x}$ = 36	CT	67.3 (I)
				70.9 (U)
Williams [122]	8	$\bar{x}$ = 6.1^a	MRI	79.46 (I)
				88.01 (U)
Williams [123]	17	$\bar{x}$ = 2^a	MRI	79.57 (I)
				87.34 (U)
Williams [69]	9^b	$\bar{x}$ = 3.3	MRI	90%^{c}
	9^d	$\bar{x}$ = 74.6		100%^{c}

Abbreviations: CSA, cross-sectional area; I, injured leg; U, uninjured leg.
^{a}Indicates time since surgical reconstruction using a semitendinosus-gracilis autograft.
^{b}Indicates subjects identified as non-copers.
^{c}CSA normalized to the uninjured limb.
^{d}Indicates subjects identified as copers.

to the CKC exercises, even though an increase in resistance during the OKC exercise produced higher strain values that were not noted during a squatting exercise. The strains produced during the OKC knee extension exercise with a 24 newton meters resistance were similar to those produce during a Lachman test using a 150 N anterior shear load. Therefore, the differences produced by the OKC and CKC exercises may not be clinically significant.

Although biomechanical studies suggest that OKC exercises may be no less safe than CKC exercises, clinical research has yet to confirm this hypothesis. Available clinical research suggests that cautiously incorporating OKC exercises into ACL rehabilitation will improve quadriceps function; thus further clinical trials are necessary to examine the safety of these exercises (Table 3) [122,123].

SUMMARY

This article highlighted approaches that may aid in the quest to restore quadriceps strength following ACL reconstruction. To maximize quadriceps strength, clinicians must incorporate strategies to retard AMI as well as innovative therapies to reduce muscle atrophy. If AMI can be minimized early following ACL injury and reconstruction, its negative consequences can be reduced and likely will lead to a more effective and efficient recovery. The best strategy to maximize quadriceps strength may be to include interventions that will target inhibition in addition to those that are focused on minimizing atrophy.

References

[1] Hurley MV, Jones DW, Wilson D, et al. Rehabilitation of quadriceps inhibition due to isolated rupture of the anterior cruciate ligament. Journal of Orthopaedic Rheumatology 1992;5:145–54.

[2] Shelbourne KD, Gray T. Anterior cruciate ligament reconstruction with autogenous patellar tendon graft followed by accelerated rehabilitation. A two- to nine-year follow-up. Am J Sports Med 1997;25:786–95.

[3] Urbach D, Nebelung W, Becker R, et al. Effects of reconstruction of the anterior cruciate ligament on voluntary activation of quadriceps femoris a prospective twitch interpolation study. J Bone Joint Surg Br 2001;83:1104–10.

[4] Eriksson E. Rehabilitation of muscle function after sport injury—major problem in sports medicine. Int J Sports Med 1981;2:1–6.

[5] Beynnon BD, Fleming BC, Johnson RJ, et al. Anterior cruciate ligament strain behavior during rehabilitation exercises in vivo. Am J Sports Med 1995;23:24–34.

[6] Chmielewski TL, Rudolph KS, Fitzgerald GK, et al. Biomechanical evidence supporting a differential response to acute ACL injury. Clin Biomech (Bristol, Avon) 2001;16:586–91.

[7] Decker MJ, Torry MR, Noonan TJ, et al. Landing adaptations after ACL reconstruction. Med Sci Sports Exerc 2002;34:1408–13.

[8] Keays SL, Bullock-Saxton J, Newcombe P, et al. The relationship between knee strength and functional stability before and after anterior cruciate ligament reconstruction. J Orthop Res 2003;21:231–7.

[9] Knoll Z, Kiss RM, Kocsis L. Gait adaptation in ACL deficient patients before and after anterior cruciate ligament reconstruction surgery. J Electromyogr Kinesiol 2004;14:287–94.

[10] Knoll Z, Kocsis L, Kiss RM. Gait patterns before and after anterior cruciate ligament reconstruction. Knee Surg Sports Traumatol Arthrosc 2004;12:7–14.

[11] Lysholm G, Gillquist J. Evaluation of knee ligament surgery results with special emphasis on use of a scoring scale. Am J Sports Med 1982;10:150–4.

[12] Petschnig R, Baron R, Albrecht M. The relationship between isokinetic quadriceps strength test and hop tests for distance and one-legged vertical jump test following anterior cruciate ligament reconstruction. J Orthop Sports Phys Ther 1998;28:23–31.

[13] Rudolph KS, Axe MJ, Buchanan TS, et al. Dynamic stability in the anterior cruciate ligament-deficient knee. Knee Surg Sports Traumatol Arthrosc 2001;9:62–71.

[14] Sekiya I, Muneta T, Ogiuchi T, et al. Significance of the single-legged hop test to the anterior cruciate ligament-reconstructed knee in relation to muscle strength and anterior laxity. Am J Sports Med 1998;26:384–8.

[15] Seto JL, Orofino AS, Morrissey MC, et al. Assessment of quadriceps/hamstring strength, knee ligament stability, functional and sports activity levels five years after anterior cruciate ligament reconstruction. Am J Sports Med 1988;16:170–80.

[16] Wojtys EM, Huston LJ. Longitudinal effects of anterior cruciate ligament injury and patellar tendon autograft reconstruction on neuromuscular performance. Am J Sports Med 2000;28:336–44.

[17] Wojtys EM, Huston LJ. Neuromuscular performance in normal and anterior cruciate ligament-deficient lower extremities. Am J Sports Med 1994;22:89–104.

[18] Anderson AF, Snyder RB, Lipscomb AB Sr. Anterior cruciate ligament reconstruction using the semitendinosus and gracilis tendons augmented by the losee iliotibial band tenodesis. A long-term study. Am J Sports Med 1994;22:620–4.

[19] Anderson AF, Dome DC, Gautam S, et al. Correlation of anthropometric measurements, strength, anterior cruciate ligament size, and intercondylar notch characteristics to sex differences in anterior cruciate ligament tear rates. Am J Sports Med 2001;29:58–66.

[20] Aune AK, Holm I, Risberg MA, et al. Four-strand hamstring tendon autograft compared with patellar tendon–bone autograft for anterior cruciate ligament reconstruction. A randomized study with two-year follow-up. Am J Sports Med 2001;29:722–8.

[21] Beard DJ, Dodd CA. Home or supervised rehabilitation following anterior cruciate ligament reconstruction: a randomized controlled trial. J Orthop Sports Phys Ther 1998;27:134–43.

[22] Beynnon BD, Johnson RJ, Fleming BC, et al. Anterior cruciate ligament replacement: comparison of bone–patellar tendon–bone grafts with two-strand hamstring grafts. A prospective, randomized study. J Bone Joint Surg Am 2002;84-A:1503–13.

[23] Boden BP, Moyer RA, Betz RR, et al. Arthroscopically assisted anterior cruciate ligament reconstruction: a follow-up study. Contemp Orthop 1990;20:187–94.

[24] Cardone CZ, Menegassi Z, Emygdio R. Isokinetic assessment of muscle strength following anterior cruciate ligament reconstruction 2004;12:173–7.

[25] Chen CH, Chen WJ, Shih CH, et al. Arthroscopic anterior cruciate ligament reconstruction with periosteum-enveloping hamstring tendon graft. Knee Surg Sports Traumatol Arthrosc 2004;12:398–405.

[26] Feller JA, Webster KE. A randomized comparison of patellar tendon and hamstring tendon anterior cruciate ligament reconstruction. Am J Sports Med 31;564–73.

[27] Giron F, Aglietti P, Cuomo P, et al. Anterior cruciate ligament reconstruciton with double-looped semitendinosus and gracilis tendon graft directly fixed to cortical bone: 5-year results. Knee Surg Sprots Traumatol Arthrosc 2005;13:81–91.

[28] Gobbi A, Mahajan S, Zanazzo M, et al. Patellar tendon versus quadrupled bone-semitendinosus anterior cruciate ligament reconstruction: a prospective clinical investigation in athletes. Arthroscopy 2003;19:592–601.

[29] Gobbi A, Tuy B, Mahajan M, et al. Quadrupled bone-semitendinosus anterior cruciate ligament reconstruction: a clinical investigation in a group of athletes. Arthroscopy 2003;19:691–9.

[30] Gokeler A, Schmalz T, Knopf E, et al. The relationship between isokinetic quadriceps strength and laxity on gait analysis parameters in anterior cruciate ligament reconstructed knees. Knee Surg Sports Traumatol Arthrosc 2003;11:372–8.

[31] Goradia VK, Grana WA, Pearson SE. Factors associated with decreased muscle strength after anterior cruciate ligament reconstruction with hamstring tendon grafts. Arthroscopy 2006;22:80.

[32] Hamada M, Shino K, Horibe S. Single-versus bi-socket anterior cruciate ligament reconstuction using autogenous multiple-stranded hamstring tendons with endoButton femoral fixation: a prospective study. Arthroscopy 2001;17:801–7.

[33] Hofmeister EP, Gillingham BL, Bathgate MB, et al. Results of anterior cruciate ligament reconstruction in the adolescent female. J Pediatr Orthop 2001;21:302–6.

[34] Jansson KA, Linko E, Sandelin J, et al. A prospective randomized study of patellar versus hamstring tendon autografts for anterior cruciate ligament reconstruction. Am J Sports Med 2003;31:12–8.

[35] Jarvela T, Kannus P, Latvala K, et al. Simple measurements in assessing muscle performance after an ACL reconstruction. Int J Sports Med 2002;23:196–201.

[36] Keays SL, Bullock-Saxton J, Keays AC. Strength and function before and after anterior cruciate ligament reconstruction. Clin Orthop Relat Res 2000;373:174–83.

[37] Keays SL, Bullock-Saxton J, Keays AC, et al. Muscle strength and function before and after anterior cruciate ligament reconstruction using semitendonosus and gracilis. Knee 2001;8:229–34.

[38] Keays SL, Bullock-Saxton JE, Keays AC, et al. A 6-year follow-up of the effect of graft site on strength, stability, range of motion, function, and joint degeneration after anterior cruciate ligament reconstruction: patellar tendon versus semitendinosus and gracilis tendon graft. Am J Sports Med 2007;35:729–39.

[39] Kobayashi A, Higuchi H, Terauchi M, et al. Muscle performance after anterior cruciate ligament reconstruction. Int Orthop 2004;28:48–51.

[40] Larkin JJ, Barber-Westin SD, et al. The effect of injury chronicity and progressive rehabilitation on single-incision arthroscopic anterior cruciate ligament reconstruction. Arthroscopy 1998;14(1):15–22.

[41] Lee S, Seong SC, Jo H, et al. Outcome of anterior cruciate ligament reconstruction using quadriceps tendon autograft. Arthroscopy 2004;20:795–802.

[42] Lephart SM, Kocher MS, Harner CD, et al. Quadriceps strength and functional capacity after anterior cruciate ligament reconstruction. Patellar tendon autograft versus allograft. Am J Sports Med 1993;21:738–43.

[43] Maeda A, Shino K, Horibe S, et al. Anterior cruciate ligament reconstruction with multi-stranded autogenous semitendinosus tendon. Am J Sports Med 1996;24:504–9.

[44] Marder RA, Raskind JR, Carroll M. Prospective evaluation of arthroscopically assisted anterior cruciate ligament reconstruction. Patellar tendon versus semitendinosus and gracilis tendons. Am J Sports Med 1991;19:478–84.

[45] McHugh MP, Tyler TF, Gleim GW, et al. Preoperative indicators of motion loss and weakness following anterior cruciate ligament reconstruction. J Orthop Sports Phys Ther 1998;27:407–11.

[46] Moisala AS, Jarvela T, Kannus P, et al. Muscle strength evaluations after ACL reconstruction. Int J Sports Med 2007;28:868–72.

[47] Natri A, Jarvinen M, Latvala K, et al. Isokinetic muscle performance after anterior cruciate ligament surgery. Long-term results and outcome-predicting factors after primary surgery and late-phase reconstruction. Int J Sports Med 1996;17:223–8.

[48] Osteras H, Augestad LB, Tondel S. Isokinetic muscle strength after anterior cruciate ligament reconstruction. Scand J Med Sci Sports 1998;8:279–82.

[49] Petersen W, Laprell H. Combined injuries of the medial collateral ligament and the anterior cruciate ligament. Early ACL reconstruction versus late ACL reconstruction. Arch Orthop Trauma Surg 1999;119:258–62.

[50] Pokar S, Wissmeyer T, Krischak G, et al. Arthroscopically assisted reconstruction of the anterior cruciate ligament with autologous patellar tendon replacement-plasty. 5 years results. Unfallchirurg 2001;104:317–24 [in German].

[51] Reat JF, Lintner DM. One- versus two-incision ACL reconstruction. A prospective, randomized study. Am J Knee Surg 1997;10:198.

[52] Rosenberg TD, Franklin JL, Baldwin GN, et al. Extensor mechanism function after patellar tendon graft harvest for anterior cruciate ligament reconstruction. Am J Sports Med 1992;20:519–25.

[53] Segawa H, Omori G, Koga Y. Long-term results of nonoperative treatment of anterior cruciate ligament injury. Knee 2001;8:5–11.

[54] Soon J, Chang P, Neo CPC, et al. Morbidity following anterior cruciate ligament reconstruction using hamstring autograft. Ann Acad Med Singapore 2004;33:214–9.

[55] Tashiro T, Kurosawa H, Kawakami A, et al. Influence of medial hamstring tendon harvest on knee flexor strength after anterior cruciate ligament reconstruction. A detailed evaluation with comparison of single- and double-tendon harvest. Am J Sports Med 2003;31:522–9.

[56] Witvrouw E, Bellemans J, Verdonk R, et al. Patellar tendon vs. doubled semitendinosus and gracilis tendon for anterior cruciate ligament reconstruction. Int Orthop 2001;25:308–11.

[57] Urbach D, Awiszus F. Impaired ability of voluntary quadriceps activation bilaterally interferes with function testing after knee injuries. A twitch interpolation study. Int J Sports Med 2002;23:231–6.

[58] Urbach D, Nebelung W, Ropke M, et al. Bilateral dysfunction of the quadriceps muscle after unilateral cruciate ligament rupture with concomitant injury central activation deficit. Unfallchirurg 2000;103:949–55 [in German].

[59] Urbach D, Nebelung W, Weiler HT, et al. Bilateral deficit of voluntary quadriceps muscle activation after unilateral ACL tear. Med Sci Sports Exerc 1999;31:1691–6.

[60] Lephart S, Perrin DH, Fu F. Relationship between selected physical characteristics and functional capacity in the anterior cruciate ligament insufficient athlete. J Orthop Sports Phys Ther 1992;16:174–81.

[61] Slemenda C, Brandt KD, Heilman DK, et al. Quadriceps weakness and osteoarthritis of the knee. Ann Intern Med 1997;127:97–104.

[62] Iles JF, Stokes M, Young A. Reflex actions of knee joint afferents during contraction of the human quadriceps. Clin Physiol 1990;10:489–500.

[63] Chmielewski TL, Stackhouse S, Axe MJ, et al. A prospective analysis of incidence and severity of quadriceps inhibition in a consecutive sample of 100 patients with complete acute anterior cruciate ligament rupture. J Orthop Res 2004;22:925–30.

[64] Snyder-Mackler L, De Luca PF, Williams PR, et al. Reflex inhibition of the quadriceps femoris muscle after injury or reconstruction of the anterior cruciate ligament. J Bone Joint Surg Am 1994;76:555–60.

[65] Snyder-Mackler L, Delitto A, Bailey SL, et al. Strength of the quadriceps femoris muscle and functional recovery after reconstruction of the anterior cruciate ligament. J Bone Joint Surg Am 1995;77:1167–73.

[66] Shelbourne KD, Nitz P. Accelerated rehabilitation after anterior cruciate ligament reconstruction. Am J Sports Med 1990;18:292–9.

[67] Elmqvist LG, Lorentzon R, Johansson C, et al. Does a torn anterior cruciate ligament lead to change in the central nervous drive of the knee extensors? Eur J Appl Physiol Occup Physiol 1988;58:203–7.

[68] Lorentzon R, Elmqvist LG, Sjostrom M, et al. Thigh musculature in relation to chronic anterior cruciate ligament tear: muscle size, morphology, and mechanical output before reconstruction. Am J Sports Med 1989;17:423–9.

[69] Williams GN, Snyder-Mackler L, Barrance PJ, et al. Quadriceps femoris muscle morphology and function after ACL injury: a differential response in copers versus noncopers. J Biomech 2005;38:685–93.

[70] Fahrer H, Rentsch HU, Gerber NJ, et al. Knee effusion and reflex inhibition of the quadriceps. A bar to effective retraining. J Bone Joint Surg Br 1988;70:635–8.

[71] Jensen K, Graf BK. The effects of knee effusion on quadriceps strength and knee intra-articular pressure. Arthroscopy 1993;9:52–6.

[72] Darton K. Long-latency spinal reflexes in humans. J Neurophysiol 1985;53:1604–18.

[73] Paintal AS. Block of conduction of mammalian myelinated nerve fibers by low temperatures. J Physiol 1965;503:691–8.

[74] Eldred E, Lindsley DF, Buchwald JS. The effect of cooling on mammalian muscle spindles. Exp Neurol 1960;2:144–57.

[75] Huber A, Suter E, Herzog W. Inhibition of the quadriceps muscles in elite male volleyball players. J Sports Sci 1998;16:281–9.

[76] Shakespeare DT. Reflex inhibition of the quadriceps after meniscectomy: lack of association with pain. Clin Physiol 1985;5:137–44.

[77] Stokes M, Shakespeare D, Sherman K, et al. Transcutaneous nerve stimulation and postmesniscectomy quadriceps inhibition. Int J Rehabil Res 1985;8:248.

[78] Hopkins JT, Ingersoll CD, Edwards JE, et al. Cryotherapy and TENS decrease arthrogenic muscle inhibition of the vastus medialis following knee joint effusion. J Athl Train 2002;37:25–32.

[79] Hopkins JT. Knee joint effusion and cryotherapy alter lower chain kinetics and muscle activity. J Athl Train 2006;41:177–84.

[80] Iles JF. Evidence for cutaneous and corticospinal modulation of presynaptic inhibition of Ia afferents from the human lower limb. J Physiol 1996;491:197–207.

[81] Palmieri RM, Tom JA, Weltman A, et al. Quadriceps arthrogenic muscle inhibition is partially mediated by a presynaptic spinal mechanism. Knee Surg Sports Traumatol Arthrosc 2005;13:370–6.

[82] Arvidsson I, Eriksson E. Postoperative TENS pain relief after knee surgery: objective evaluation. Orthopedics 1986;9:1346–51.

[83] Hassan BS, Doherty SA, Mockett S, et al. Effect of pain reduction on postural sway, proprioception, and quadriceps strength in subjects with knee osteoarthritis. Ann Rheum Dis 2002;61:422–8.

[84] Arvidsson I, Eriksson E, Knutsson E, et al. Reduction of pain inhibition on voluntary muscle activation by epidural analgesia. Orthopedics 1986;9:1415–9.

[85] Agostinucci J. The effect of topical anesthetics on skin sensation and soleus motoneuron reflex excitability. Arch Phys Med Rehabil 1994;75:1233–40.

[86] Agostinucci J, Powers WR. Motoneuron excitability modulation after desensitization of the skin by iontophoresis of lidocaine hydrochloride. Arch Phys Med Rehabil 1992;73:190–4.

[87] Binder-Macleod SA, Halden EE, Jungles KA. Effects of stimulation intensity on the physiological responses of human motor units. Med Sci Sports Exerc 1995;27:556–65.

[88] Cabric M, Appel HJ, Resic A. Fine structural changes in electrostimulated human skeletal muscle. Evidence for predominant effects on fast muscle fibres. Eur J Appl Physiol Occup Physiol 1987;57:1–5.

[89] Trimble MH, Enoka RM. Mechanism underlying the training effects associated with neuromuscular electrical stimulation. Phys Ther 1991;71:273–80.

[90] Delitto AS, Rose J, Mckowen JM, et al. Electrical stimulation versus voluntary exercise in strengthening thigh musculature after anterior cruciate ligament surgery. Phys Ther 1988;71:455–64.

[91] Eriksson E, Haggmark T. Comparison of isometric muscle training and electrical stimulation supplementing isometric muscle training in the recovery after major knee ligament surgery. Am J Sports Med 1979;7:169–71.

[92] Fitzgerald GK, Piva SR, Irrgang JJ. A modified neuromuscular electrical stimulation protocol for quadriceps strength training following anterior cruciate ligament reconstruction. J Orthop Sports Phys Ther 2003;33:492–501.

[93] Snyder-Mackler L, Delitto A, Stralka S, et al. Use of electrical stimulation to enhance recovery of quadriceps femoris muscle force production in patients following anterior cruciate ligament reconstruction. Phys Ther 1994;74:901–7.

[94] Snyder-Mackler L, Ladin L, Schepsis AA, et al. Electrical stimulation of the thigh muscles after reconstruction of the anterior cruciate ligament. J Bone Joint Surg Am 1991;73:1025–36.

[95] Wigerstad-Lossing I, Grimby G, Jonsson T, et al. Effects of electrical muscle stimulation combined with voluntary contractions after knee ligament surgery. Med Sci Sports Exerc 1988;20:93–8.

[96] Stevens JE, Mizner RL, Snyder-Mackler L. Neuromuscular electrical stimulation for quadriceps muscle strengthening after bilateral total knee arthroplasty: a case series. J Orthop Sports Phys Ther 2004;34:21–9.

[97] Dursun N, Dursun E, Kilic Z. Electromyographic biofeedback-controlled exercise versus conservative care for patellofemoral pain syndrome. Arch Phys Med Rehabil 2001;82:1692–5.

[98] Draper V. Electromyographic biofeedback and recovery of quadriceps femoris muscle function following anterior cruciate ligament reconstruction. Phys Ther 1990;70:11–7.

[99] Draper V, Ballard L. Electrical stimulation versus electromyographic biofeedback in the recovery of quadriceps femoris muscle function following anterior cruciate ligament surgery. Phys Ther 1991;71:455–61.

[100] Ingersoll CD, Knight KL. Patellar location changes following EMG biofeedback or progressive resistive exercises. Med Sci Sports Exerc 1991;23:1122–7.

[101] Krebs DE. Clinical electromyographic feedback following meniscectomy. A multiple regression experimental analysis. Phys Ther 1981;61:1017–21.

[102] Thompson B, Geller NL, Hunsberger S, et al. Behavioral and pharmacologic interventions: the Raynaud's Treatment Study. Control Clin Trials 1999;20:52–63.

[103] Wannstedt G, Craik RL. Clinical evaluation of a sensory feedback device: the limb load monitor. Bull Prosthet Res 1978;8–49.

[104] Basmajian JV. Control and training of individual motor units. Science 1963;141:440–1.

[105] Maitland ME, Ajemian SV, Suter E. Quadriceps femoris and hamstring muscle function in a person with an unstable knee. Phys Ther 1999;79:66–75.

[106] Lindstedt SL, LaStayo PC, Reich TE. When active muscles lengthen: properties and consequences of eccentric contractions. News Physiol Sci 2001;16:256–61.

[107] Hortobagyi T, Barrier J, Beard D, et al. Greater initial adaptations to submaximal muscle lengthening than maximal shortening. J Appl Physiol 1996;81:1677–82.

[108] Hortobagyi T, Hill JP, Houmard JA, et al. Adaptive responses to muscle lengthening and shortening in humans. J Appl Physiol 1996;80:765–72.

[109] LaStayo PC, Pierotti DJ, Pifer J, et al. Eccentric ergometry: increases in locomotor muscle size and strength at low training intensities. Am J Physiol Regul Integr Comp Physiol 2000;278:R1281–8.

[110] LaStayo PC, Ewy GA, Pierotti DD, et al. The positive effects of negative work: increased muscle strength and decreased fall risk in a fail elderly population. J Gerontol A Biol Sci Med Sci 2003;58:M419–24.

[111] Dibble LE, Hale T, Marcus RL, et al. The safety and feasibility of high-force eccentric resistance exercise in persons with Parkinson's disease. Arch Phys Med Rehabil 2006;87:1280–2.

[112] Dibble LE, Hale TF, Marcus RL, et al. High-intensity resistance training amplifies muscle hypertrophy and functional gains in persons with Parkinson's disease. Mov Disord 2006;21:1444–52.

[113] Gerber JP, Marcus RL, Dibble LE, et al. Effects of early progressive eccentric exercise on muscle structure after anterior cruciate ligament reconstruction. J Bone Joint Surg Am 2007;89:559–70.

[114] Gerber JP, Marcus RL, Dibble LE, et al. Safety, feasibility, and efficacy of negative work exercise via eccentric muscle activity following anterior cruciate ligament reconstruction. J Orthop Sports Phys Ther 2007;37:10–8.

[115] Gerber JP, Marcus RL, Dibble LE, et al. Early application of negative work via eccentric ergometry following anterior cruciate ligament reconstruction: a case report. J Orthop Sports Phys Ther 2006;36:298–307.

[116] Bynum EB, Barrack RL, Alexander AH. Open versus closed chain kinetic exercises after anterior cruciate ligament reconstruction. A prospective randomized study. Am J Sports Med 1995;23:401–6.

[117] Mikkelsen C, Werner S, Eriksson E. Closed kinetic chain alone compared to combined open and closed kinetic chain exercises for quadriceps strengthening after anterior cruciate ligament reconstruction with respect to return to sports: a prospective matched follow-up study. Knee Surg Sports Traumatol Arthrosc 2000;8:337–42.

[118] Tagesson S, Oberg B, Good L, et al. A comprehensive rehabilitation program with quadriceps strengthening in closed versus open kinetic chain exercise in patients with anterior cruciate ligament deficiency: a randomized clinical trial evaluating dynamic tibial translation and muscle function. Am J Sports Med 2008;36:298–307.

[119] Heijne A, Werner S. Early versus late start of open kinetic chain quadriceps exercises after ACL reconstruction with patellar tendon or hamstring grafts: a prospective randomized outcome study. Knee Surg Sports Traumatol Arthrosc 2007;15:402–14.

[120] Perry MC, Morrissey MC, King JB, et al. Effects of closed versus open kinetic chain knee extensor resistance training on knee laxity and leg function in patients during the 8- to 14-week postoperative period after anterior cruciate ligament reconstruction. Knee Surg Sports Traumatol Arthrosc 2005;13:357–69.

[121] Beynnon BD, Fleming BC. Anterior cruciate ligament strain in vivo: a review of previous work. J Biomech 1998;31:519–25.

[122] Williams GN, Barrance PJ, Snyder-Mackler L, et al. Altered quadriceps control in people with anterior cruciate ligament deficiency. Med Sci Sports Exerc 2004;36:1089–97.

[123] Williams GN, Snyder-Mackler L, Barrance PJ, et al. Neuromuscular function after anterior cruciate ligament reconstruction with autologous semitendinosus–gracilis graft. J Electromyogr Kinesiol 2005;15:170–80.

Clin Sports Med 27 (2008) 425–448

CLINICS IN SPORTS MEDICINE

ELSEVIER
SAUNDERS

Trunk and Hip Control Neuromuscular Training for the Prevention of Knee Joint Injury

Gregory D. Myer, MS, CSCS[a,b,*],
Donald A. Chu, PhD, PT, ATC, CSCS[b,c,d],
Jensen L. Brent, BS, CSCS[a,d],
Timothy E. Hewett, PhD, FACSM[a,e]

[a]Sports Medicine Biodynamics Center and Human Performance Laboratory Cincinnati Children's Hospital Medical Center, Cincinnati Children's Hospital, 3333 Burnet Avenue; MLC 10001, Cincinnati, OH 45229, USA
[b]Rocky Mountain University of Health Professions, 561 East 1860 South, Provo, UT 84606, USA
[c]Athercare Fitness and Rehabilitation Clinic, 200 Basiniside Way, Alameda, CA 94502, USA
[d]Ohlone College, Newark, CA 94560-4902, USA
[e]Departments of Pediatrics, Orthopaedic Surgery, College of Medicine and the Departments of Biomedical Engineering and Rehabilitation Sciences, University of Cincinnati, 231Albert Sabin Way, Cincinnati, OH 45267, USA

Female athletes are currently reported to be four to six times more likely to sustain a sports-related noncontact anterior cruciate ligament (ACL) injury than male athletes in comparable high-risk sports [1–4]. Altered or decreased neuromuscular control during the execution of sports movements, which manifests itself in resultant lower limb joint mechanics (motions and loads), may increase the risk of ACL injury in female athletes [5–10]. The established links between lower limb mechanics and noncontact ACL injury risk led to the development of neuromuscular training interventions designed to prevent ACL injury by targeting deficits identified in specific populations [7,10–15]. Injury prevention protocols have resulted in positive preventative and biomechanical changes in female athletic populations at high risk for knee injury [12,14,16,17]. Pilot work also indicates that female athletes categorized as high risk for ACL injury, based on previous coupled biomechanical and epidemiologic studies [7], may be more responsive to neuromuscular training [11]. Yet, following neuromuscular training, the high-risk categorized females may

The authors would like to acknowledge funding support from National Institutes of Health/NIAMS Grant R01-AR049735 and R01-AR055563.

*Corresponding author. Cincinnati Children's Hospital, 3333 Burnet Avenue; MLC 10001, Cincinnati, OH 45229. E-mail address: greg.myer@cchmc.org (G.D. Myer).

0278-5919/08/$ – see front matter
doi:10.1016/j.csm.2008.02.006

Published by Elsevier Inc.
sportsmed.theclinics.com

not reduce risk predictors to levels similar to those of low-risk categorized athletes [11]. In addition, Agel and colleagues [18] performed a 13-year (1989-2002) retrospective epidemiologic study to determine the trends in ACL injury rates of National Collegiate Athletic Association soccer and basketball athletes. These authors reported significant decreases in ACL injuries in male soccer players, whereas female soccer athletes showed no change over the same time period. Both female basketball and soccer players showed no change in the rates of noncontact ACL injuries over the study period, and the magnitude of difference in rates (3.6 X) between their male counterparts remained unchanged [18].

There is evidence that neuromuscular training not only reduces the levels of potential biomechanical risk factors for ACL injury, but also decreases knee and ACL injury incidence in female athletes [12]. Reevaluation of ACL injury rates in female athletes, however, indicates that this important health issue has yet to be resolved [18]. The purpose of this article is to provide evidence to outline a novel theory used to define the mechanisms related to increased risk of ACL injury in female athletes. In addition, this discussion will include theoretical constructs for the description of the mechanisms that lead to increased risk. Finally, a clinical application section will outline neuromuscular training techniques designed to target deficits that underlie the proposed mechanism of increased risk of knee injury in female athletes.

BIOMECHANICS RELATED TO INCREASED RISK OF ANTERIOR CRUCIATE LIGAMENT INJURY IN FEMALE ATHLETES

Altered or decreased neuromuscular control during the execution of sports movements, which result in excessive resultant lower limb joint motions and loads, may increase risk of ACL injury in female athletes [7]. Hewett and colleagues [7] prospectively demonstrated that measures of lower extremity valgus, including knee abduction motion and torque, during jump-landing tasks, predicted ACL injury risk in young female athletes with high sensitivity and specificity. Females also exhibit increased lower extremity valgus alignment and load compared with males during landing and pivoting movements [5,9,19–26]. Females often demonstrate similar lower extremity valgus alignments at the time of injury [27–29]. Although the understanding of the biomechanics associated with ACL injuries that predict increased injury risk is important, it may be more relevant to define the mechanisms that actually induce the high-risk biomechanics. If this is determined, more effective and efficient neuromuscular intervention could be made available to high-risk female populations.

THE RELATIONSHIP OF GROWTH AND MATURATION TO DEVELOPMENT OF HIGH-RISK MECHANISMS

Contrary to the findings of sex differences in ACL injury risk in the adolescent female athlete, there is no evidence that a sex difference in ACL injury rates is present in prepubescent athletes [30–33]. Although knee injuries do occur in the preadolescent athlete, with up to 63% of the sports-related injuries in children aged 6 to 12 years reported as joint sprains, and with the majority of these sprains occurring at the knee [33], specific sprains such as injuries to the anterior cruciate ligament are more rare. Additionally, sex differences do not appear to be present in children before their growth spurt [30–32]. Following their growth spurt, however, female athletes have higher rates of sprains than males, and this trend continues into maturity [34].

During peak height velocity in pubertal athletes, the tibia and femur grow at relatively rapid rates in both sexes [35]. Rapid growth of the two longest levers in the human body initiate height increases and, in turn, an increased height of the center of mass, making muscular control of trunk more difficult. In addition, increased body mass, concomitant with growth of joint levers, may initiate greater joint forces that are more difficult to balance and dampen during high-velocity maneuvers [21,36,37]. Thus, it can be hypothesized that following the onset of puberty and the initiation of peak height velocity, increased tibia and femur lever length, with increased body mass and height of the center of mass, in the absence of increases in strength and recruitment of the musculature at the hip and trunk, lead to decreased core stability or control of trunk motion during dynamic tasks [38]. As female athletes reach maturity, decreased core stability may underlie their tendency to demonstrate increased dynamic lower extremity valgus load (hip adduction and knee abduction) during dynamic tasks (Fig. 1) [21,36,37,39–41].

The authors have developed a concept of trunk and lower extremity function that identifies the body's core as a critical modulator of lower extremity alignments and loads during dynamic tasks. The trunk and hip stabilizers may preactivate to counterbalance trunk motion and regulate lower extremity postures [39–41]. Reduced preactivation of the trunk and hip stabilizers may allow increased lateral trunk positions that can incite knee abduction loads [42]. Decreased core stability and muscular synergism of the trunk and hip stabilizers may affect performance in power activities and may increase the incidence of injury secondary to lack of control of the center of mass, especially in female athletes [43,44]. Zazulak and colleagues [45] reported that factors related to core stability predicted risk of knee injuries in female athletes but not in male athletes. Thus, the current evidence indicates that compromised function of the trunk and hip stabilizers, as they relate to core neuromuscular control, may underlie the mechanisms of increased ACL injury risk in female athletes [7,27,28,45].

NEUROMUSCULAR TRAINING TARGETED TO THE TRUNK

Table 1 presents a neuromuscular training protocol to be instituted with female athletes to target deficits in trunk and hip control [46]. Five exercise phases are used to facilitate progressions designed to improve the athlete's ability to control the trunk and improve core stability during dynamic activities (Table 1). All exercises in each phase progressively increase the intensity of the exercise

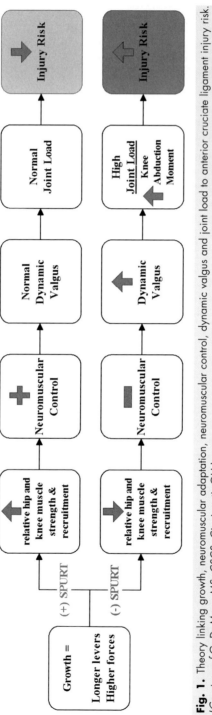

Fig. 1. Theory linking growth, neuromuscular adaptation, neuromuscular control, dynamic valgus and joint load to anterior cruciate ligament injury risk. (*Courtesy of* G. D. Myer, MS, CSCS, Cincinnati, OH.)

Table 1
Suggested repetitions and sets of the selected exercise progressions

Progression 1	Time	Reps	Sets	
Lateral Jump and Hold		8		
Step-Hold		8	R	L
BOSU (Round) Supermans		10		
BOSU (Round) Double Knee-Hold	20 secs			
Single Leg Lateral Airex Hop-Hold		4	R	L
Single Tuck Jump-Soft Landing		10		
Front Lunges		10	R	L
Lunge Jumps	10 secs		R	L
BOSU (Flat) Double Leg Pelvic Bridges		10		
Single Leg 90° Hop-Hold		8	R	L
BOSU (Round) Lateral Crunch		10	R	L
Box Double Crunch		15		
Swiss Ball Back Hyperextensions		15		
Progression 2	**Time**	**Reps**	**Sets**	
Lateral Jumps	10 secs			
Jump-Single Leg Hold		8	R	L
BOSU (Round) Toe Touch Swimmers		10	R	L
BOSU (Round) Single Knee-Hold	20 secs		R	L
Single Leg Lateral BOSU (Round) Hop-Hold		8	R	L
Double Tuck Jump		6		
Walking Lunges		10		
Scissor Jumps	10 secs			
BOSU (Flat) Single Leg Pelvic Bridges		10	R	L
Single Leg 90° Airex Hop-Hold		8	R	L
Box Lateral Crunch		10	R	L
Box Swivel Double Crunch		15	R	L
Swiss Ball Back Hyperextensions with Ball Reach		15		
Progression 3	**Time**	**Reps**	**Sets**	
Lateral Hop and Hold		8	R	L
Hop-Hold		8	R	L
Prone Bridge (Elbows and Knees) Hip Extension opposite shoulder flexion		10		
Swiss Ball Bilateral Kneel	20 secs			
Single Leg Lateral BOSU (Round) Hop-Hold with Ball Catch		4	R	L
Repeated Tuck Jump	10 secs			
Walking Lunges Unilateraly Weighted		10	R	L
Lunge Jumps Unilateraly Weighted	10 secs		R	L
BOSU (Flat) Single Leg Pelvic Bridges with Ball Hold		10	R	L
Single Leg 90° Airex Hop-Hold Reaction Ball Catch		6	R	L
BOSU (Round) Lateral Crunch with Ball Catch		8	R	L
BOSU (Round) Swivel Ball Touches (Feet up)		15		
Swiss Ball Hyperextensions with Back Fly		15		

Table 1
(continued)

Progression 4	Time	Reps	Sets	
Lateral Hops	10 secs		R	L
Hop-Hop-Hold		8	R	L
Prone Bridge (Elbows and toes) Hip Extension		10	R	L
Swiss Ball Bilateral Kneel with Partner Pertubations	20 secs			
Single Leg 4 Way BOSU (Round) Hop-Hold		3 cycles	R	L
Side to Side Barrier Tuck Jumps	10 secs			
Walking Lunges with Plate Cross-over		10	R	L
Scissor Jumps Unilateraly Weighted	10 secs		R	L
Supine Swiss Ball Hamstring Curl		10		
Single Leg 180° Airex Hop-Hold		8	R	L
Swiss Ball Lateral Crunch		15	R	L
BOSU (Round) Double Crunch		15		
Swiss Ball Hyperextensions with Ball Reach Lateral		15	R	L
Progression 5	Time	Reps	Sets	
X-hops		6 cycles	R	L
Crossover-Hop-Hop-Hold		8	R	L
Prone Bridge (Elbows and toes) Hip Extension opposite shoulder flexion		10	R	L
Swiss Ball Bilateral Kneel with Lateral Ball Catch	20 secs			
Single Leg 4 Way BOSU (Round) Hop-Hold with Ball Catch		3 cycles	R	L
Side to Side Reaction Barrier Tuck Jumps	10 secs			
Walking Lunges with Unilateral Shoulder Press		10	R	L
Scissor Jumps with Ball Swivel	10 secs		R	L
Swivel Russian Hamstring Curl		10		
Single Leg 180° Airex Hop-Hold Reaction Ball Catch		8	R	L
Swiss Ball Lateral Crunch with Ball Catch		8	R	L
BOSU (Round) Swivel Double Crunch		15	R	L
Swiss Ball Hyperextensions with Lateral Ball Catch		15		

techniques. End-stage progressions incorporate lateral trunk perturbations that force the athlete to decelerate and control the trunk in the coronal plane to successfully execute the prescribed technique. Selected protocol sets and repetitions should only be soft guidelines that can provide an attainable goal for the athlete (see Table 1). Initial volume selection should be low to allow the athlete the opportunity to learn to perform the exercises with excellent technique and relative ease. Volume (or resistance, when applicable) should be increased until the athlete can perform all of the exercises at the prescribed volume and intensity with near-perfect technique. The individual supervising the athletes should be skilled in recognizing the proper technique for a given exercise, and should encourage the athlete to maintain proper technique. If the athlete fatigues to a point that she can no longer perform the exercise with near-perfect form, or she displays a sharp decline in proficiency, then she should be instructed to stop. The repetitions for each completed exercise should be noted, and the goal of the next training session should be to continue to improve technique and to increase volume (number of repetitions) or intensity (resistance). Once an athlete becomes proficient with all exercises within a progression phase, she can advance to the next successive phase. To improve exercise techniques, instructors should give continuous and immediate feedback to the young athlete, both during and after each exercise bout. This will make the athlete aware of proper form and technique, as well as undesirable and potentially dangerous positions. All of the exercises selected for the initial phase before progression are adapted from previous epidemiologic or interventional investigations that have reported reductions in ACL injury risk or risk factors (Table 2) [47–50]. The protocol progressions were developed from previous biomechanical investigations that reported reductions in knee abduction load in female athletes following their training protocols [10,11,13,14]. The novelty to this training approach is that the current protocol will incorporate exercises that perturb the trunk to improve control of trunk and improve core stability and decrease the mechanisms that induce high knee abduction loading in female athletes.

EFFECTS OF TRUNK NEUROMUSCULAR TRAINING ON HIP ABDUCTION PEAK TORQUE

Pilot studies that used the proposed neuromuscular training targeted to the trunk (TNMT) protocol indicate that increased standing hip abduction strength can be improved in female athletes (Tables 3–15) [46]. Hip abduction strength and recruitment may improve the ability of female athletes to increase control of lower extremity alignment and decrease knee abduction motion and loads resulting from increased trunk displacement during sports activities. Future investigations are needed to determine if improved hip strength following

Table 2	
Exercise progressions and the published intervention from which it was derived and adapted	
Trunk- and hip-focused exercise progressions	Exercise adapted from intervention
Lateral jumping progression	Hewett 1999, Mandelbaum 2004
Single-leg anterior progression	Hewett 1999
Prone trunk stability progression	Myer 2007
Kneeling trunk stability progression	Myer 2007
Single-leg lateral progression	Myklebust 2003, Petersen 2006
Tuck jump progression	Hewett 1999
Lunge progression	Mandelbaum 2004
Lunge jump progression	Hewett 1999
Hamstring-specific progression	Mandelbaum 2004
Single-leg rotatory progression	Myklebust 2003, Petersen 2006
Lateral trunk progression	Myer 2007
Trunk flexion progression	Myklebust 2003, Petersen 2006
Trunk extension progression	Myer 2007

Table 3
Lateral jumping progression

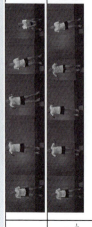

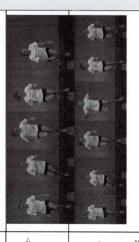

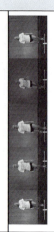

Phase 1—Lateral jump and hold

The athlete prepares for this exercise by standing with her feet close together and her knees slightly bent. The athlete should jump laterally over a line, keeping her knees bent and staying close to the line. When she lands on the opposite side, she should descend into a deep hold immediately.

Phase 2—Lateral jumps

The athlete prepares for this exercise by standing with her feet close together and knees slightly bent on one side of the line. The athlete should jump sideways over the line, keeping her knees bent and staying close to the line. When the athlete lands on the opposite side, she should redirect back to the initial position immediately. The athlete should repeat this sequence as quickly as she can while maintaining proper form. When teaching this exercise, encourage the athlete to achieve as many repetitions as possible in the allotted time by jumping close to the lines, shortening the ground contact time, and not using excessive height on the jumps. Do not allow the athlete to perform a double hop on the side of the line. Early in the training, the athlete may focus on the line; as her technique improves, encourage her to shift her visual focus away from the line to outside cues.

Phase 3—Lateral hop and hold

The athlete prepares for this exercise by standing on one foot with her knee slightly bent. The athlete should jump sideways over a line, keeping her knee bent and staying close to the line. When she lands on the opposite side, she should descend into a single-leg deep hold immediately.

Phase 4—Lateral hops

The athlete prepares for this exercise by standing on one leg with her knee slightly bent on one side of the line. The athlete should jump sideways over the line, keeping her knee bent and staying close to the line. When the athlete lands on the opposite side, she should redirect back to the initial position immediately. When teaching this exercise, encourage the athlete to achieve as many repetitions as possible in the allotted time by jumping close to the lines, shortening the ground contact time, and not using excessive height on the jumps. Do not allow the athlete to perform a double hop on the side of the line. Early in the training the athlete may focus on line; as her technique improves encourage her to shift her visual focus away from the line to outside cues.

Phases 5–10—Hops

The athlete begins facing a quadrant pattern standing on a single limb with her support knee slightly bent. She will hop diagonally, landing in the opposite quadrant, maintaining forward stance, and holding the deep knee flexion landing for 3 seconds. The athlete then hops laterally into the side quadrant, again holding the landing. Next, the athlete will hop diagonally backward holding the landing. Finally, she hops laterally into the initial quadrant holding the landing. The athlete should repeat this figure 8 pattern for the required number of sets. Encourage the athlete to maintain balance during each landing, keeping her eyes up and her focus away from her feet.

Table 4
Single-leg anterior progression

Phase 1—Step-hold
The athlete starts by taking a quick step forward and continues by balancing in a deep hold position on the leg onto which she stepped.

Phase 2—Jump–single-leg hold
The athlete will begin this exercise in the athletic position. The athlete proceeds to jump forward, landing and balancing on one leg in a deep hold position.

Phase 3—Hop hold
Starting in a balanced position on one foot, the athlete hops forward, landing and balancing on one leg in a deep hold position.

Phase 4—Hop-hop-hold
The athlete hops forward twice quickly, landing and balancing on one leg in a deep hold position.

Phase V—Crossover hop-hop-hold
The athlete hops forward while alternating legs three times quickly, landing and balancing on one leg in a deep hold position.

Adapted from Myer G, Brent J, Ford K, et al. A pilot study to determine the effect of trunk and hip focused neuromuscular training on hip and knee isokinetic strength. Br J Sports Med 2008. Epub ahead of print. doi:10.1136/bjsm.2007.046086; with permission.

Table 5
Prone trunk stability progression

Phase 1—BOSU (round) toe touch swimmers

The athlete begins in a prone position with her abdomen centered on the round side of the BOSU and her arms overhead and legs extended. The athlete reaches back with one arm to touch opposite foot and returns to the outstretched superman position.

Phase 2—BOSU (round) swimmers with partner perturbations

The athlete begins in prone position with abdomen centered on the round side of the BOSU and with her arms overhead and legs extended. The movement is initiated by elevating the opposite arm and leg, and held for 3 seconds. A partner will offer random perturbations by stepping on different sides of the BOSU during the exercise.

Phase 3—Prone bridge (elbows and knees) hip extension opposed shoulder flexion

The athlete begins in prone position with her elbows flexed and balanced on an Airex pad and knees on the ground. The movement is initiated by elevating the opposite arm and leg, and held for a single count and finished by returning to the original position.

Phase 4—Prone bridge (elbows and toes) hip extension

The athlete begins in prone position with elbows flexed and balanced on an Airex pad and toes on the ground. The movement is initiated by elevating the each leg individually, held for a single count, and finished by re-turning to the original position.

Phase 5—Prone bridge (elbows and toes) hip extension opposite shoulder flexion

The athlete begins in prone position with elbows flexed and balanced on an Airex pad and toes on the ground. The movement is initiated by elevating the opposite arm and leg, held for a single count, and fin-ished by returning to the original position.

Adapted from Myer G, Brent J, Ford K, et al. A pilot study to determine the effect of trunk and hip focused neuromuscular training on hip and knee isokinetic strength. Br J Sports Med 2008. Epub ahead of print. doi:10.1136/bjsm.2007.046086; with permission.

Table 6
Kneeling trunk stability progression

Phase 1—BOSU (round) double-knee hold

The athlete begins this exercise by balancing in a kneeling position with her knees on each side of the round side of the BOSU. The athlete will maintain this balanced position with the hips slightly flexed for the duration of the exercise.

Phase 2—BOSU (round) single-knee hold

The athlete begins this exercise by balancing in a kneeling position with one knee directly in the middle of the round side of the BOSU and the other knee extended out to the side. The athlete will maintain this balanced position with the hip slightly flexed for the duration of the exercise.

Phase 3—Swiss ball bilateral kneel

The athlete kneels and balances on Swiss ball with feet off the ground. A spotter should be available at all times in front of the athlete.

Phase 4—Swiss ball bilateral kneel with partner perturbations

The athlete kneels and balances on Swiss ball with her feet off of the ground. Once the athlete is stabilized, a partner can perturb the ball by kicking in unanticipated directions. A spotter should be available at all times in front of the athlete.

Phase 5—Swiss ball bilateral kneel with lateral ball catch

The athlete kneels and balances on Swiss ball with feet off the ground. A ball should be tossed back and forth with a partner to increase the difficulty of this exercise.

Table 7
Single-leg lateral progression

Phase 1—Single-leg lateral Airex hop hold
Athlete starts on one side of the Airex pad and hops laterally onto the Airex. The athlete should maintain balance and hold the knee in a flexed position. The athlete then hops off the other side of the Airex onto the ground, maintains balance, and then repeats the exercise in the other direction.

Phase 2—Single-leg lateral BOSU (round) hop hold
Athlete starts on one side of the BOSU and hops laterally onto the BOSU. The athlete should maintain balance and hold the knee in a flexed position. The athlete then hops off the other side of the BOSU onto the ground, maintains balance, and then repeats the exercise in the other direction.

Phase 3—Single-leg lateral BOSU (Round) hop hold with ball catch
The athlete starts on one side of the BOSU and hops laterally onto the BOSU. The athlete should maintain balance and hold the knee in a flexed position. The athlete then hops off the other side of the BOSU onto the ground, maintains balance, and then repeats the exercise in the other direction. The athlete is challenged further by having to catch and return a ball upon each landing.

Phase 4—Single-leg four-way BOSU (round) hop hold
The athlete starts in a single-leg athletic position immediately behind the BOSU. The athlete hops forward onto the round side of the BOSU and lands in a balanced position. After achieving a balanced single leg stance on the BOSU, the athlete proceeds to hop off the BOSU laterally and assumes this same stance on the floor immediately next to the BOSU. The athlete then will continue to hop on and off the BOSU, achieving a balanced athletic position, in each of the four directions: forward, backward, lateral, and medial.

Phase 5—Single-leg four-way BOSU (round) hop hold with ball catch
The athlete starts in a single-leg athletic position immediately behind the BOSU. The athlete hops forward onto the round side of the BOSU and lands in a balanced position. After achieving a balanced single-leg stance on the BOSU, the athlete proceeds to hop off the BOSU laterally and assumes this same stance on the floor immediately next to the BOSU. The athlete then will continue to hop on and off the BOSU, achieving a balanced athletic position, in each of the four directions: forward, backward, lateral, and medial. A ball should be tossed back and forth with a partner upon landing to increase the difficulty of this exercise.

Table 8
Tuck jump progression

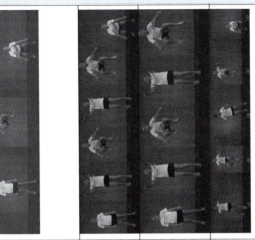

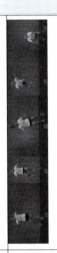

Phase 1—Single tuck jump soft landing

The athlete starts in the athletic position with her feet shoulder width apart. The athlete initiates a vertical jump with a slight crouch downward while she extends her arms behind her. The athlete then swings her arms forward as she simultaneously jumps straight up and pulls her knees up as high as possible. At the highest point of the jump the athlete should be positioned in the air with her thighs parallel to the ground. On landing, the athlete should land softly, using a toe to midfoot rocker landing. The athlete should not continue this jump if she cannot control the high landing force or keep her knees aligned during landing. If the athlete is unable to raise the knees to the proper height, it may be valuable to instruct her to grasp the knees and then bring the thighs to horizontal.

Phase 2—Double tuck jump

Similar to the single tuck jump but with an additional jump performed immediately after the first jump. The athlete should focus on maintaining good form and minimizing time on the ground between jumps.

Phase 3—Repeated tuck jump

The athlete starts in the athletic position with her feet shoulder width apart. The athlete initiates a vertical jump with a slight crouch downward while she extends her arms behind her. The athlete then swings her arms forward as she simultaneously jumps straight up and pulls her knees up as high as possible. At the highest point of the jump, the athlete should be positioned in the air with her thighs parallel to the ground. When landing, the athlete immediately should begin the next tuck jump.

Phase 4—Side-to-side tuck jumps

The athlete starts in the athletic position with her feet shoulder width apart. The athlete initiates a vertical jump over a barrier with a slight crouch downward while she extends her arms behind her. The athlete then swings her arms forward as she simultaneously jumps straight up and pulls her knees up as high as possible. At the highest point of the jump, the athlete should be positioned in the air with her thighs parallel to the ground. When landing, the athlete immediately should begin the next tuck jump back to the other side of the barrier.

Phase 5—Side-to-side reaction barrier tuck jumps

The athlete starts in the athletic position with her feet shoulder width apart. The athlete initiates a vertical jump over a barrier with a slight crouch downward while she extends her arms behind her. The athlete then swings her arms forward as she simultaneously jumps straight up and pulls her knees up as high as possible. At the highest point of the jump, the athlete should be positioned in the air with her thighs parallel to the ground. When landing, the athlete immediately should begin the next tuck jump. When prompted, the athlete should jump to the other side of the barrier without breaking rhythm.

Table 9
Lunge progression

Phase 1—Front lunges

The athlete begins by stepping forward from a standing position. The step should be exaggerated in length to the point that her front leg is positioned with the knee flexed to 90° and the lower leg completely vertical. The back leg should be as straight as possible and the torso upright. Emphasis should be placed on getting the hips as low as possible while maintaining the previously described body position. Driving off the front leg and returning to the original position complete the exercise.

Phase 2—Walking lunges

The athlete performs a lunge, and instead of returning to the start position she steps through with the back limb and proceeds forward with a lunge on the opposite limb. Encourage the athlete to lunge her front limb far enough out so that her knee does not advance beyond her ankle during the exercise. An alternative coaching method is to instruct the athlete to attempt to maintain a constant low center of gravity and roll through the lunges. This increases the intensity of the exercise and attempts to mimic motions frequently occurring in sports.

Phase 3—Walking lunges unilaterally weighted

The athlete performs a lunge, and instead of returning to the start position, she steps through with the back limb and proceeds forward with a lunge on the opposite limb while holding a dumbbell in one hand. Encourage the athlete to lunge her front limb far enough out so that her knee does not advance beyond her ankle during the exercise. This exercise is repeated with the dumbbell in the opposite hand.

Phase 4—Walking lunges with plate crossover

The athlete performs a lunge, and instead of returning to the start position, she steps through with the back limb and proceeds forward with a lunge on the opposite limb while reaching with a weight plate to the open side of the body. Encourage the athlete to lunge her front limb far enough out so that her knee does not advance beyond her ankle during the exercise.

Phase 5—Walking lunges with unilateral shoulder press

The athlete performs a lunge, and instead of returning to the start position, she steps through with the back limb and proceeds forward with a lunge on the opposite limb while pressing a dumbbell above her head. The weight should move up and down with the same tempo and direction as the lunge. Encourage the athlete to lunge her front limb far enough out so that her knee does not advance beyond her ankle during the exercise.

Table 10
Lunge jump progression

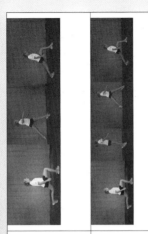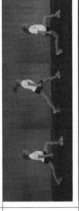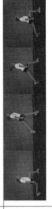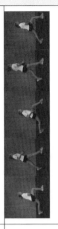

Phase 1—Lunge jumps

The athlete starts in an extended stride position with the hips pushed forward, and the front knee positioned directly above the ankle and flexed to 90°. The back leg is fully extended at the hip and knee providing minimal support for the stance. The athlete should jump vertically off of the front support leg, maintaining the starting position during flight and landing. The jump is repeated as quickly as possible while still achieving maximum vertical height. To coach this jump, encourage the athlete to keep the back leg straight and use it only for balance support. The front leg obtains vertical power. Stance support percentages are approximately 80% for the front leg and 20% for the back.

Phase 2—Scissor jumps

The athlete starts in an extended stride position with the hips pushed forward, and the front knee positioned directly above the ankle and flexed to 90°. The back leg is fully extended at the hip and knee providing minimal support for the stance. The athlete should jump vertically off of the front support leg and switch the position of the legs while in flight. The jump is repeated as quickly as possible while still achieving maximum vertical height. The athlete will be jumping off alternate legs on each jump during this exercise.

Phase 3—Lunge jumps unilaterally weighted

The athlete starts in an extended stride position with her hips pushed forward, and the front knee positioned directly above the ankle and flexed to 90°. The back leg is extended fully at the hip and knee providing minimal support for the stance. The athlete should jump vertically off of the front support leg, maintaining the starting position during flight and landing. The jump is repeated as quickly as possible while still achieving maximum vertical height. To unilaterally weight this exercise, a dumbbell should be held in one hand. This exercise then is repeated with the dumbbell in the opposite hand.

Phase 4—Scissor jumps unilaterally weighted

The athlete starts in an extended stride position with the hips pushed forward, and the front knee positioned directly above the ankle and flexed to 90°. The back leg is extended fully at the hip and knee providing minimal support for the stance. The athlete should jump vertically off of the front support leg and switch the position of the legs while in flight. The jump is repeated as quickly as possible, while still achieving maximum vertical height. To unilaterally weight this exercise, a dumbbell should be held in one hand. The athlete will be jumping off alternate legs on each jump during this exercise. This exercise is repeated with the dumbbell in the opposite hand.

Phase 5—Scissor jumps with ball swivel

The athlete starts in an extended stride position with the hips pushed forward, and the front knee positioned directly above the ankle and flexed to 90°. The back leg is extended fully at the hip and knee providing minimal support for the stance. The athlete should jump vertically off of the front support leg and switch the position of the legs while in flight. The jump is repeated as quickly as possible while still achieving maximum vertical height. To unilaterally weight this exercise, a medicine ball should be swiveled to the open side of the body during each jump. The athlete will be jumping off alternate legs.

Table 11
Hamstring-specific progression

Phase 1—BOSU (flat) pelvic bridge

The athlete lays supine with her hip and knees flexed and her feet planted on the flat side of the BOSU. The athlete then extends her hips and elevates her trunk off the ground to execute a pelvic bridge. This position should be held for 3 seconds before repeating the next repetition.

Phase 2—BOSU (flat) single-leg pelvic bridge

The athlete lays supine with her hip and knees flexed and a single foot planted on the flat side of the BOSU and the contralateral leg fully extended. The athlete then extends her hips and elevates her trunk off the ground to execute a pelvic bridge. This position should be held for 3 seconds before repeating the next repetition.

Phase 3—BOSU (flat) single leg pelvic bridge

The athlete lays supine with her hip and knees flexed and a single foot planted on the flat side of the BOSU and the contralateral leg fully extended holding a ball directly above her in her hands. The athlete then extends her hips and elevates her trunk off the ground to execute a pelvic bridge. This position should be held for 3 seconds before repeating the next repetition. A weight plate is positioned on the hips to add resistance.

Phase 4—Supine Swiss ball hamstring curl

The athlete lays supine with her hip and knees flexed with both heels planted on top of a Swiss ball. The athlete then extends her hips and elevates her trunk off the ground while pulling her heels in to her buttocks.

Phase 5—Russian hamstring curl with lateral touch

The athlete begins in a kneeling position with a partner providing foot support and torso support (with band assistance). The athlete extends at the knee to lower her torso toward the ground. Once touching the BOSU with her chest, the athlete swivels her trunk and returns to the original position. The coach should provide enough assistance so that the exercise can be performed without flexing at the hip.

Table 12
Single-leg rotatory progression

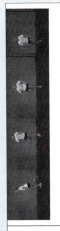
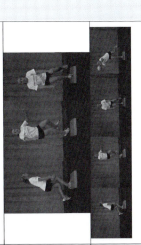
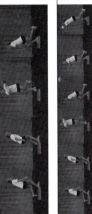
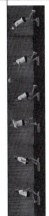

Phase 1—Single-leg 90° hop hold

The starting position for this jump is with the athlete in a semicrouched position on the single limb being trained. The jump should focus on attaining maximum height while maintaining good form upon landing. During the flight phase, the athlete should rotate 90°. The landing occurs on the same leg and should be performed with deep knee flexion (to 90°). The landing should be held for a minimum of 3 seconds to be counted as a successful landing. Coach this jump with care to protect the athlete from injury. Start the athlete with a submaximal effort so she can experience the difficulty of the jump. Continue to increase the intensity of the jump as the athlete improves her ability to stick and hold the final landing. Have the athlete keep her focus away from her feet, to help prevent too much forward lean.

Phase 2—Single-leg 90° Airex hop hold

The starting position for this jump is with the athlete in a semicrouched position on the single limb being trained. The jump should focus on attaining maximum height while maintaining good form upon landing. During the flight phase, the athlete should rotate 90°. The landing occurs on the same leg and should be performed with deep knee flexion (to 90°). The landing should be held for a minimum of 3 seconds on an Airex pad to be counted as a successful landing. Coach this jump with care to protect the athlete from injury.

Phase 3—Single-leg 90° hop-hold reaction ball catch

The starting position for this jump is with the athlete in a semicrouched position on the single limb being trained. The jump should focus on attaining maximum height while maintaining good form upon landing. During the flight phase, the athlete should rotate 90°. The landing occurs on the same leg and should be performed with deep knee flexion (to 90°). The landing should be held for a minimum of 3 seconds on an Airex pad to be counted as a successful landing. Upon landing a ball will be passed back and forth with the athlete to increase the difficulty of a successful landing.

Phase 4—Single-leg 180° Airex hop hold

The starting position for this jump is with the athlete in a semicrouched position on the single limb being trained. The jump should focus on attaining maximum height while maintaining good form upon landing. During the flight phase, the athlete should rotate 180°. The landing occurs on the same leg and should be performed with deep knee flexion (to 90°). The landing should be held for a minimum of 3 seconds on an Airex pad to be counted as a successful landing.

Phase 5—Single-leg 180° Airex hop-hold reaction ball catch

The starting position for this jump is with the athlete in a semicrouched position on the single limb being trained. The jump should focus on attaining maximum height while maintaining good form upon landing. During the flight phase, the athlete should rotate 180°. The landing occurs on the same leg and should be performed with deep knee flexion (to 90°). The landing should be held for a minimum of 3 seconds on an Airex pad to be counted as a successful landing. Upon landing, a ball will be passed back and forth with the athlete to increase the difficulty of a successful landing.

Table 13
Lateral trunk progression

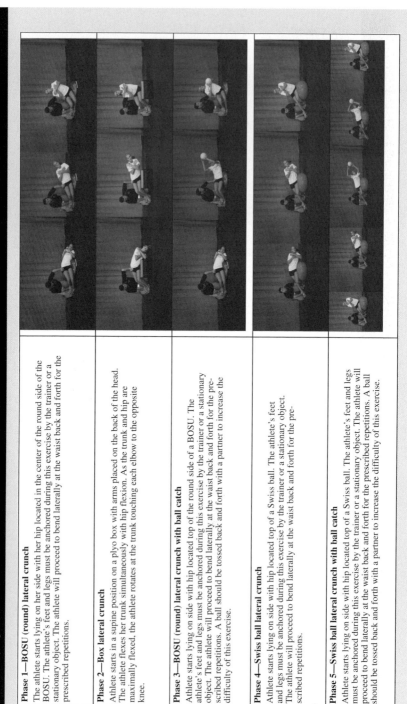

Phase 1—BOSU (round) lateral crunch

The athlete starts lying on her side with her hip located in the center of the round side of the BOSU. The athlete's feet and legs must be anchored during this exercise by the trainer or a stationary object. The athlete will proceed to bend laterally at the waist back and forth for the prescribed repetitions.

Phase 2—Box lateral crunch

Athlete starts in a supine position on a plyo box with arms placed on the back of the head. The athlete flexes her trunk simultaneously with hip flexion. As the trunk and hip are maximally flexed, the athlete rotates at the trunk touching each elbow to the opposite knee.

Phase 3—BOSU (round) lateral crunch with ball catch

Athlete starts lying on side with hip located top of the round side of a BOSU. The athlete's feet and legs must be anchored during this exercise by the trainer or a stationary object. The athlete will proceed to bend laterally at the waist back and forth for the pre-scribed repetitions. A ball should be tossed back and forth with a partner to increase the difficulty of this exercise.

Phase 4—Swiss ball lateral crunch

Athlete starts lying on side with hip located top of a Swiss ball. The athlete's feet and legs must be anchored during this exercise by the trainer or a stationary object. The athlete will proceed to bend laterally at the waist back and forth for the pre-scribed repetitions.

Phase 5—Swiss ball lateral crunch with ball catch

Athlete starts lying on side with hip located top of a Swiss ball. The athlete's feet and legs must be anchored during this exercise by the trainer or a stationary object. The athlete will proceed to bend laterally at the waist back and forth for the prescribed repetitions. A ball should be tossed back and forth with a partner to increase the difficulty of this exercise.

Table 14
Trunk flexion progression

Phase 1—Box double crunch

The athlete starts out supine on a plyometric box or similar object and flexes her trunk simultaneous with hip flexion.

Phase 2—Box swivel double crunch

Athlete starts in a supine position on a plyo box with arms placed across chest. The athlete flexes her trunk simultaneous with hip flexion. As the trunk and hip are maximally flexed, the athlete rotates at the trunk, touching each elbow to the opposite knee.

Phase 3—BOSU (round) swivel ball touches (feet up)

Athlete starts sitting on the round side of a BOSU holding a medicine ball. The athlete will proceed to swivel at the trunk to touch the medicine ball to the floor for each repetition.

Phase 4—BOSU (round) double crunch

Athlete starts sitting on the round side of a BOSU. The athlete flexes her trunk simultaneous with hip flexion.

Phase 5—BOSU (round) swivel double crunch

Athlete starts sitting on the round side of a BOSU. The athlete flexes her trunk simultaneous with hip flexion. As the trunk and hip are maximally flexed, the athlete rotates at the trunk touching each elbow to the opposite knee.

Table 15
Trunk extension progression

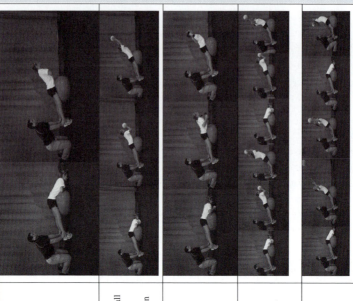

Phase 1—Swiss ball back hyperextensions

The athlete begins in a prone position on the Swiss ball, with her hips centered on top of the Swiss ball and a partner anchoring her feet to the floor. The movement is initiated by extending her hips and lower back to bring the athlete into a position of slight hyperextension. The position should be maintained for a short pause and then returned to the flexed position.

Phase 2—Swiss ball back hyperextensions with ball reach

The athlete begins in a prone position on the Swiss ball with her hips centered on top of the Swiss ball and a partner anchoring her feet to the floor. The movement is initiated by extending hips and lower back to bring the athlete into a position of slight hyperextension. While performing this motion the athlete will also extend and return a medicine ball from the chest to full shoulder and elbow extension and back to the chest.

Phase 3—Swiss ball hyperextensions with back fly

The athlete begins in a prone position on the Swiss ball with her hips centered on top of the Swiss ball and a partner anchoring her feet to the floor. The movement is initiated by extending hips and lower back to bring the athlete into a position of slight hyperextension. The position should be maintained while the athlete brings dumbbells out to the side similar to a back fly exercise.

Phase 4—Swiss ball hyperextensions with ball reach lateral

The athlete begins in a prone position on the Swiss ball with her hips centered on top of the Swiss ball and a partner anchoring her feet to the floor. The movement is initiated by extending hips and lower back to bring the athlete into a position of slight hyperextension. The position should be maintained while the athlete brings a medicine ball above her head and slightly to the side.

Phase 5—Swiss ball hyperextensions with lateral ball catch

The athlete begins in a prone position on the Swiss ball with her hips centered on top of the Swiss ball and a partner anchoring her feet to the floor. The movement is initiated by extending hips and lower back to bring the athlete into a position of slight hyperextension. The position should be maintained while the athlete brings a medicine ball above her head and slightly to the side. A ball should be tossed back and forth with a partner to increase the difficulty of this exercise.

TNMT translates into reduced knee abduction load in high ACL injury risk female athletes. If this association is observed, then parallel investigations should be undertaken to determine if TNMT is effective in pubertal and pre-pubertal athletes to artificially induce neuromuscular spurt (defined as the natural adaptation of increased power, strength, and coordination that occur with increasing chronologic age and maturational stage in adolescent boys), especially related to relative hip strength and control, which often reduced are as young female athletes mature [15,51].

SUMMARY

Dynamic neuromuscular analysis-oriented training appears to reduce ACL injuries in adolescent and mature female athletes [17,47,49,50]. Targeted neuromuscular training, at or near the onset of puberty, simultaneously may improve lower extremity strength and power, reduce dangerous biomechanics related to ACL injury risk, and improve single-leg balance [21,52]. Neuromuscular training could be advocated in pre- and early pubertal children to help prevent the development of high-risk knee joint biomechanics that develop during this stage of maturation [53]. A preemptive approach that institutes early interventional training also may reduce the peak rate of ACL injuries that occurs near age 16 in young girls [54]. Because of the near 100% risk of osteoarthritis in the ACL injured population [55], with or without surgical reconstruction, prevention is the only effective intervention for these life-altering injuries. Additional efforts toward the development of more specific injury prevention protocols targeted toward the mechanism demonstrated in high-risk athletes with the determination of the timing of when these interventions should most effectively be used is imperative. Specifically, neuromuscular training that focuses on trunk control instituted just before pubertal development may provide the most effective interventional approach to alleviate high-risk biomechanics in female athletes.

Acknowledgements

The authors would like to thank the Mason School Volleyball Program, especially head coach Tiann Keesling, and Mason School Athletic Director Scott Stemple, Principal Dr. Dave Allen, and Superintendent Kevin Bright for their support to this project.

References

[1] Arendt E, Dick R. Knee injury patterns among men and women in collegiate basketball and soccer. NCAA data and review of literature. Am J Sports Med 1995;23(6):694–701.

[2] Malone TR, Hardaker WT, Garrett WE, et al. Relationship of gender to anterior cruciate ligament injuries in intercollegiate basketball players. J South Orthop Assoc 1993;2(1):36–9.

[3] Myklebust G, Maehlum S, Holm I, et al. A prospective cohort study of anterior cruciate ligament injuries in elite Norwegian team handball. Scand J Med Sci Sports 1998;8(3): 149–53.

[4] Mihata LC, Beutler AI, Boden BP. Comparing the incidence of anterior cruciate ligament injury in collegiate lacrosse, soccer, and basketball players: implications for anterior cruciate ligament mechanism and prevention. Am J Sports Med 2006;34(6):899–904.

[5] Ford KR, Myer GD, Hewett TE. Valgus knee motion during landing in high school female and male basketball players. Med Sci Sports Exerc 2003;35(10):1745–50.

[6] Ford KR, Myer GD, Toms HE, et al. Gender differences in the kinematics of unanticipated cutting in young athletes. Med Sci Sports Exerc 2005;37(1):124–9.

[7] Hewett TE, Myer GD, Ford KR, et al. Biomechanical measures of neuromuscular control and valgus loading of the knee predict anterior cruciate ligament injury risk in female athletes: a prospective study. Am J Sports Med 2005;33(4):492–501.

[8] McLean SG, Lipfert SW, van den Bogert AJ. Effect of gender and defensive opponent on the biomechanics of sidestep cutting. Med Sci Sports Exerc 2004;36(6):1008–16.

[9] Chappell JD, Yu B, Kirkendall DT, et al. A comparison of knee kinetics between male and female recreational athletes in stop–jump tasks. Am J Sports Med 2002;30(2):261–7.

[10] Myer GD, Ford KR, McLean SG, et al. The effects of plyometric versus dynamic stabilization and balance training on lower extremity biomechanics. Am J Sports Med 2006;34(3):490–8.

[11] Myer GD, Ford KR, Brent JL, et al. Differential neuromuscular training effects on ACL injury risk factors in "high-risk" versus "low-risk" athletes. BMC Musculoskelet Disord 2007; 8(39):1–7.

[12] Hewett TE, Ford KR, Myer GD. Anterior cruciate ligament injuries in female athletes: part 2, a meta-analysis of neuromuscular interventions aimed at injury prevention. Am J Sports Med 2006;34(3):490–8.

[13] Myer GD, Ford KR, Brent JL, et al. The effects of plyometric versus dynamic balance training on power, balance and landing force in female athletes. J Strength Cond Res 2006;20(2): 345–53.

[14] Myer GD, Ford KR, Palumbo JP, et al. Neuromuscular training improves performance and lower-extremity biomechanics in female athletes. J Strength Cond Res 2005;19(1):51–60.

[15] Myer GD, Ford KR, Hewett TE. Rationale and clinical techniques for anterior cruciate ligament injury prevention among female athletes. J Athl Train 2004;39(4):352–64.

[16] Myer GD, Ford KR, Brent JL, et al. The effects of plyometric versus dynamic balance training on landing force and center of pressure stabilization in female athletes. Br J Sports Med 2005;39(6):397.

[17] Hewett TE, Lindenfeld TN, Riccobene JV, et al. The effect of neuromuscular training on the incidence of knee injury in female athletes. A prospective study. Am J Sports Med 1999;27(6):699–706.

[18] Agel J, Arendt EA, Bershadsky B. Anterior cruciate ligament injury in national collegiate athletic association basketball and soccer: a 13-year review. Am J Sports Med 2005;33(4): 524–30.

[19] Ford KR, Myer GD, Smith RL, et al. A comparison of dynamic coronal plane excursion between matched male and female athletes when performing single leg landings. Clin Biomech 2006;21(1):33–40.

[20] Malinzak RA, Colby SM, Kirkendall DT, et al. A comparison of knee joint motion patterns between men and women in selected athletic tasks. Clin Biomech 2001;16(5):438–45.

[21] Hewett TE, Myer GD, Ford KR. Decrease in neuromuscular control about the knee with maturation in female athletes. J Bone Joint Surg Am 2004;86-A(8):1601–8.

[22] McLean SG, Huang X, Su A, et al. Sagittal plane biomechanics cannot injure the ACL during sidestep cutting. Clin Biomech 2004;19:828–38.

[23] Kernozek TW, Torry MR, VH H, et al. Gender differences in frontal and sagittal plane biomechanics during drop landings. Med Sci Sports Exerc 2005;37(6):1003–12 [discussion: 1013].

[24] Zeller BL, McCrory JL, Kibler WB, et al. Differences in kinematics and electromyographic activity between men and women during the single-legged squat. Am J Sports Med 2003;31(3):449–56.

[25] Pappas E, Hagins M, Sheikhzadeh A, et al. Biomechanical differences between unilateral and bilateral landings from a jump: gender differences. Clin J Sport Med 2007;17(4): 263–8.

[26] Hewett TE, Ford KR, Myer GD, et al. Gender differences in hip adduction motion and torque during a single leg agility maneuver. J Orthop Res 2006;24(3):416–21.

[27] Olsen OE, Myklebust G, Engebretsen L, et al. Injury mechanisms for anterior cruciate ligament injuries in team handball: a systematic video analysis. Am J Sports Med 2004;32(4):1002–12.

[28] Krosshaug T, Nakamae A, Boden BP, et al. Mechanisms of anterior cruciate ligament injury in basketball: video analysis of 39 cases. Am J Sports Med 2007;35(3):359–67.

[29] Boden BP, Dean GS, Feagin JA, et al. Mechanisms of anterior cruciate ligament injury. Orthopedics 2000;23(6):573–8.

[30] Andrish JT. Anterior cruciate ligament injuries in the skeletally immature patient. Am J Orthop 2001;30(2):103–10.

[31] Buehler-Yund C. A longitudinal study of injury rates and risk factors in 5- to 12-year-old soccer players. Cincinnati (OH): Environmental health, University of Cincinnati; 1999.

[32] Clanton TO, DeLee JC, Sanders B, et al. Knee ligament injuries in children. J Bone Joint Surg Am 1979;61(8):1195–201.

[33] Gallagher SS, Finison K, Guyer B, et al. The incidence of injuries among 87,000 Massachusetts children and adolescents: results of the 1980–81 Statewide Childhood Injury Prevention Program Surveillance System. Am J Public Health 1984;74(12):1340–7.

[34] Tursz A, Crost M. Sports-related injuries in children. A study of their characteristics, frequency, and severity, with comparison to other types of accidental injuries. Am J Sports Med 1986;14(4):294–9.

[35] Tanner JM, Davies PS. Clinical longitudinal standards for height and height velocity for North American children. J Pediatr 1985;107(3):317–29.

[36] Hewett TE, Myer GD, Ford KR, et al. Preparticipation physical exam using a box drop vertical jump test in young athletes: the effects of puberty and sex. Clin J Sport Med 2006;16(4):298–304.

[37] Hewett TE, Biro FM, McLean SG, et al. Identifying female athletes at high risk for ACL Injury. Cincinnati Children's Hospital, National Institutes of Health; 2003.

[38] Ford KR, Myer GD, Hewett TE. Increased trunk motion in female athletes compared to males during single-leg landing. Med Sci Sports Exerc 2007;39(5):S70.

[39] Wilson JD, Dougherty CP, Ireland ML, et al. Core stability and its relationship to lower extremity function and injury. J Am Acad Orthop Surg 2005;13:316–25.

[40] Hodges PW, Richardson CA. Contraction of the abdominal muscles associated with movement of the lower limb. Phys Ther 1997;77(2):132–42 [discussion: 142–134].

[41] Hodges PW, Richardson CA. Feedforward contraction of transversus abdominis is not influenced by the direction of arm movement. Exp Brain Res 1997;114(2):362–70.

[42] Winter DA. Biomechanics and motor control of human movement. 3rd edition. New York: John Wiley & Sons, Inc.; 2005.

[43] Ireland ML. The female ACL: why is it more prone to injury? Orthop Clin North Am 2002;33(4):637–51.

[44] Zatsiorsky VM. Science and practice of strength training. Champaign (IL): Human Kinetics; 1995.

[45] Zazulak BT, Hewett TE, Reeves NP, et al. The effects of core proprioception on knee injury: a prospective biomechanical–epidemiological study. Am J Sports Med 2007;35(3):368–73.

[46] Myer GD, Brent JL, Ford KR, et al. A pilot study to determine the effect of trunk and hip focused neuromuscular training on hip and knee isokinetic strength. British Journal of Sports Medicine, Epub March 4, 2008.

[47] Mandelbaum BR, Silvers HJ, Watanabe D, et al. Effectiveness of a neuromuscular and proprioceptive training program in preventing the incidence of ACL injuries in female athletes: two-year follow up. Am J Sports Med 2005;33(6):1003–10.

[48] Hewett TE, Stroupe AL, Nance TA, et al. Plyometric training in female athletes. Decreased impact forces and increased hamstring torques. Am J Sports Med 1996;24(6):765–73.

[49] Petersen W, Braun C, Bock W, et al. A controlled prospective case control study of a prevention training program in female team handball players: the German experience. Arch Orthop Trauma Surg 2006;125(9):614–21.

[50] Myklebust G, Engebretsen L, Braekken IH, et al. Prevention of anterior cruciate ligament injuries in female team handball players: a prospective intervention study over three seasons. Clin J Sport Med 2003;13(2):71–8.

[51] Brent JL, Myer GD, Ford KR, et al. A longitudinal examination of hip abduction strength in adolescent males and females. Med Sci Sports Exerc 2008;39(5).

[52] Myer GD, Ford KR, Divine JG, et al. Specialized dynamic neuromuscular training can be utilized to induce neuromuscular spurt in female athletes. Med Sci Sports Exerc 2004;36(5):343–4.

[53] Ford KR, Myer GD, Divine JG, et al. Landing differences in high school female soccer players grouped by age. Med Sci Sports Exerc 2004;36(5):S293.

[54] Shea KG, Pfeiffer R, Wang JH, et al. Anterior cruciate ligament injury in pediatric and adolescent soccer players: an analysis of insurance data. J Pediatr Orthop 2004;24(6):623–8.

[55] Myklebust G, Bahr R. Return-to-play guidelines after anterior cruciate ligament surgery. Br J Sports Med 2005;39(3):127–31.

Clin Sports Med 27 (2008) 449–462

CLINICS IN SPORTS MEDICINE

ELSEVIER
SAUNDERS

Neuromuscular Consequences of Low Back Pain and Core Dysfunction

Robert R. Hammill, MA, ATC[a],
James R. Beazell, PT, DPT, OCS, FAAOMPT, ATC[b],
Joseph M. Hart, PhD, ATC[c],*

[a]Health and Exercise Science, Bridgewater College, 402 East College Street,
Box 166, Bridgewater, VA 22812, USA
[b]University of Virginia-Healthsouth, 545 Ray C. Hunt Drive, Suite 210, PO Box 800105,
Charlottesville, VA 22903, USA
[c]Department of Orthopaedic Surgery, University of Virginia, 400 Ray C. Hunt Drive,
Suite 330, PO Box 800159, Charlottesville, VA 22908, USA

Low back pain (LBP) remains a significant health care issue with reportedly over 50% prevalence in the general population and over 70% likely to experience at least one episode of LBP during in their lifetime [1,2]. The annual incidence has been estimated to involve almost half of the population, resulting in over $40 billion in economic costs in the form of medical treatment and lost wages [3,4]. The social and economic impact of LBP is evident in the literature and in practice. Considering the high prevalence of LBP, it is not surprising that 2% of the United States workforce are compensated for back injuries each year [4], suggesting an enormous economic burden reaching $25 billion annually [5].

The prevalence of nonspecific LBP may vary because of vague diagnostic and research-based definitions of nonspecific LBP and the myriad of possible etiologies and associated comorbidities [6,7]. Regardless of these issues, nonspecific LBP presents a major clinical problem because of the likelihood of high cost [5], limited activity levels [8], and recurrence [9]. Recurrent episodes, particularly those that cause modified or limited activity levels in people who choose to or who must remain active.

LBP that does not require surgical intervention presents a clinical dilemma for the treating physicians and therapists. Nonspecific LBP has been defined as a recurring, benign, and self-limiting condition [10], but it causes considerable pain for patients and reduced quality of life, demanding a multidisciplinary treatment strategy. Although many treatment strategies for nonspecific LBP have been studied at length, the recurrent nature of nonspecific LBP suggests that optimal and most effective treatment strategies have yet to be defined

*Corresponding author. E-mail address: joehart@virginia.edu (J.M. Hart).

0278-5919/08/$ – see front matter
doi:10.1016/j.csm.2008.02.005

clearly. It is important for clinicians to progress through a careful process of evaluation and ruling out to reach the appropriate diagnosis and make appropriate treatment recommendations. An understanding of underlying structural and neuromuscular components contributing to the development of LBP and the consequences of such injury in active individuals warrants consideration when developing treatment strategies.

This article discusses neuromuscular deficits that are present in people who have LBP. Additionally, it discusses how stability of the lumbar, pelvic, and hip regions (collectively called the core) contributes to neuromuscular deficits in people who have LBP.

SUBJECTIVE MEASURES OF LOW BACK PAIN SEVERITY

The Oswestry Disability Index (ODI) originally was presented in the literature in 1980 in a small sample [11] and later modified [12]. Its current form functions to identify disturbances in activities of daily living caused by LBP. The ODI was developed to define low back disability and thus assess changes associated with treatment of an LBP population. It is the most commonly used functional outcome questionnaire, representing an estimated 59% of all randomized control trials that use similar tools [13]. The original study used only 25 participants, and each was retested within 24 hours. Despite the confounding changes that can occur in a symptomatic population over time, excellent reliability has been reported for its one day test–retest reliability [14], with naturally reduced reliability for retest after 1 week [15].

To complete the ODI, subjects rate their disability caused by LBP in 10 categories (pain intensity, personal care, lifting, walking, sitting, standing, sleeping, social life, traveling, and homemaking/employment). Some versions include a question about sex life instead of homemaking/employment. Numeric values are assigned to the disability description that is selected by the subject/patient, where low scores indicate less perceived disability, and high scores indicate greater disability. The total score is tallied and normalized to a percentage, where smaller percentages indicate less disability. Scores under 20% indicate minimal functional disability; 20% to 40% scores indicate moderate disability, and 40%–60% scores indicate a severe disability [11]. People who have chronic LBP, and people without low back pain have been compared using the ODI. A weighted mean of 43.3 for chronic LBP sufferers and 10.2 for people without low back pain has been reported previously [16]. Therefore it is possible for a person to perceive disability according to the ODI without having a history.

The Roland-Morris Disability Questionnaire (RDQ) is a measure of health status relative to disability caused by LBP [17]. The RDQ lists 24 statements regarding disability caused by LBP. Subjects/patients select which statements pertain to them (ie, which statements they perceive to be true for them at the time they are completing the questionnaire). The range of scores is 0 to 24, with 0 indicating no disability. The test–retest reliability originally was reported to be very good (r = .91) if administered on the same day, with reduced reliability over time [18], and it is sensitive to changes in patients' LBP [19].

A complete side-by-side comparison of the ODI and RDQ has been presented previously [20].

Both the ODI and RDQ are short, simple surveys that are effective in describing current state and changes in disability caused by LBP. In previous research, subject/patient interview/history-taking has been used to identify patients who have recurring LBP. For example, people reporting more than three episodes of LBP in the past year and/or more than five lifetime episodes have been identified as a group with a history of recurring episodes of LBP, where an episode of LBP was defined as that which causes a limitation or modification to daily, routine activities [21–23]. People who have recurrent LBP according to these criteria and who report to be recreationally active have been found to respond differently following fatiguing lumbar paraspinal exercise [21–24]. Proper identification of LBP for research purposes is of utmost importance and may differ based on the research question and study design. For example, the subjective rating scale may need to match the primary outcome of the study. Although the ODI may work well for a young and active population, quantifying the number of previous episodes of LBP has successfully identified neuromuscular differences compared with healthy control subjects (average age of low back pain subjects was approximately 22 years) [21,23]. No specific subjective rating scale, however, has been developed and validated for a young and athletic population.

RISK FOR DEVELOPING LOW BACK PAIN

The etiology of chronic low back dysfunction has been described as 70% from internal disc disruption, zygapophyseal (facet) joint pain, and sacroiliac joint pain [25]. LBP has been attributed to sacroiliac joint dysfunction, accounting for up to 15% of LBP [25]. Ten percent to 40% of LBP cases arise from lumbar facet joints [26]; however, LBP arising from a combination of disc and facet joint is rare [27]. The relative contribution of the sacrococcygeal joint is not well-reported in the literature; however, it has been proposed that dysfunction of the coccyx also can contribute to LBP [28].

The likelihood of experiencing LBP increases with age, where the peak prevalence of LBP occurs in people aged 55 to 64 years in the United States but seems to cause the greatest level of activity level limitations in persons younger than 45 years [4,29]. The likelihood of experiencing LBP also increases with time, where lifetime prevalence is highest, indicating 85% to 90% of the population are likely to experience an episode of LBP in their lifetime, and about 2% to 5% of the population report experiencing an episode of back pain at least once every year [30–32]. A person who has an episode of recurrent LBP experiences a 60% to 70% recovery rate by 6 weeks and a 80% to 90% recovery rate by 12 weeks following onset [4]. Residual LBP symptoms and recurrence, however, are common. Longer-duration LBP may reduce the likelihood of returning to work or activity considerably [4]. Lengthy durations of LBP symptoms also reduce the likelihood of recovery. Patients reporting symptoms for more than 6 months have 50% chance of returning to work and may never experience pain-free periods of uninterrupted work greater than 2 years [33]. This suggests that recurrent LBP and chronic LBP considerably limit functional ability and may have a profound effect on quality of life.

Previous LBP seems to be the best predictor for the likelihood of experiencing a future episode of LBP [34,35]. Physical and biological measures, however, also have proven valuable tools for predicting LBP. Weakness and imbalances in the muscles that surround the hips, spine, and pelvis [36–38]; poor abdominal muscle endurance [39]; hamstring tightness [39–41]; poor spinal flexibility [39,41]; and reduced lumbar lordosis [41] are associated with risk for developing episodes of LBP. Although it is likely that a different combination of factors influences the development of each episode of LBP, recurring episodes pose a major clinical dilemma because of the risk for chronic disability. Therefore, recurrent, nonspecific and nonsurgical LBP presents a challenge to the surgical or rehabilitation team, because pinpointing an underlying cause is extremely difficult.

Panjabi [42] has put forth the concept of clinical instability. This is not instability that an orthopedist would have to treat surgically but a lack of segmental control of the lumbar spine. An intricate interplay between the osseo-ligamentous system, the myofascial system, and the neural control system works together to provide stability to the lumbar spine and surrounding areas such as the hips and pelvis. Disruption in any of these systems will lead to a lack of segmental control. The ability to maintain the spinal segment in a neutral zone is important for maintaining overall stability and preventing spinal pain. Stability of most joints in the body is maintained by a combination of the different tissues including the osseo-ligamentous system, muscular system, and the neuromuscular system [42–46]. The ability of the patient to maintain an efficient coordination between these systems will allow him or her to function without undue stress on other systems.

LOW BACK PAIN AND CORE STABILITY

Practitioners have been inundated for some time now regarding the importance of the core. The core of the body has been identified as the structures about the lumbo-pelvic-hip complex [47]. Active and passive structures in this area provide dynamic and static stability to this area of the body, which provides an essential base for appendicular movement. Core stability is instantaneous and relies heavily on muscular capacity (ie, endurance) and neuromuscular control [48]. An intricate relationship between these factors provides core stability and allows for appropriate control of movement and positioning of the trunk over the pelvis and legs [49] during activity, which, in turn, provides a stable base for extremity movement and efficient absorption of forces transmitted through the extremities during complex multijoint activities.

There is a distinction between muscles that provide gross movement and those that provide intrinsic stability of the various segments of the spine. Bergmark [50] suggested that most muscles that act on the trunk can be categorized into local or global divisions. The local division can be defined as those muscles that act locally, typically across just one or two joints, and function to provide segmental stability [50]. Conversely, the global division may be defined as muscles that act to provide gross motion and contribute very little to segmental stability [50].

Recent literature supports the theory that recurrent, nonspecific LBP is the result of inefficient neuromuscular control of the transverse abdominus muscle [51–53]. The integrity of the muscle tissue is not faulty, but the way people who have LBP plan movements is not effective. The transverse abdominus muscle should become more active before the prime mover of any limb. In people who have LBP, this is not the case. Essentially, the way a person with LBP prepares for movement is at fault [51–53]. In the presence of inappropriate and/or aberrant muscle activity caused by poor core stability, potentially detrimental body positions and neuromuscular adaptations may prevail as the person who has LBP continues with activities of daily living because of necessity or persistence. These adaptations may explain the recurrent nature of LBP and may be discouraging to the LBP sufferer, resulting in modified or limited activity levels. Inappropriate neuromuscular or positional adaptations also may expose joint surfaces to excessive and unusual forces, thereby exposing to further injury local to the site of dysfunction (ie, the core) and ultimately reduce quality of life.

NEUROMUSCULAR CHARACTERISTICS OF PERSONS WITH LOW BACK PAIN

Panjabi [54] presented three subsystems for spinal stability. Ligaments and bones comprise the passive subsystem; muscle makes up the active subsystem, and the nervous tissue serves as the control subsystem (Fig. 1). Function of the control subsystem in the neutral zone of the spine's range of motion [43,44] is

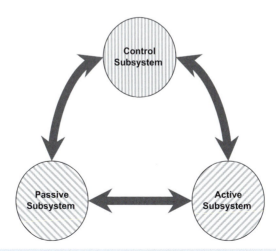

Fig. 1. Panjabi's theoretic model of the three subsystems associated with control of the spine. (*Data from* Panjabi MM. The stabilizing system of the spine. Part II. Neutral zone and instability hypothesis. J Spinal Disord 1992;5(4):390–6. Panjabi MM.) The stabilizing system of the spine. Part I. Function, dysfunction, adaptation, and enhancement. J Spinal Disord 1992;5(4):383–9.

HAMMILL, BEAZELL, & HART

integral to preventing LBP. It is at this neutral zone in the range of motion where the passive structures (passive subsystem) of the spine contribute little to each segment's stability [55]. Faulty control of the deep local muscles may lead to a back injury or recurrence [55,56].

Nonspecific LBP often is attributed to weak abdominal musculature. Although this may be true, a mass of evidence points toward a faulty motor program. The literature indicates that a preactivation of the transverse abdominus before peripheral movements of the upper [52,57] or lower extremity [52] occurs in healthy people (without low back pain). The fact that some of the stabilizing muscles of the trunk are activated in a feed-forward fashion suggests they play an integral role in the performance of peripheral movements and protecting the spine in preparation for movement. In the case of subjects who have LBP, the transverse abdominus muscle does not activate in advance [43]. This delay may put stress on the passive structures of the spine and pelvis at the initiation of movement, as the spinal segments and pelvis are not being influenced by dynamic or static stabilizers.

The intervertebral joints of the lumbar spine require a cocontraction for stability [58]. In normal stance, the lumbar segments are in an open-packed position because of the lack of passive restraint at this point in space. This point in space where lumbar segments have no passive restraints acting on them has been termed the neutral zone [59] and requires muscle contraction to stabilize. The lumbar vertebrae and pelvic girdle can be stabilized effectively by cocontracting the transverse abdominus and multifidus muscles [60–63]. This technique may be valuable for two reasons. One, it will increase intra-abdominal pressure, thereby stabilizing the lumbar segments [60] and, two, it may compress the sacroiliac joints [64]. Other muscles may contribute to sacroiliac joint stability. These muscles include the gluteus maximus, erector spinae, biceps femoris, and latissimus dorsi [58], but the extent to which each of these contributes the stability of the sacroiliac joint remains speculative.

Conversely, cocontractions of the superficial abdominal musculature (ie, the rectus abdominus and external obliques) also may provide significant stability to lumbar segments, but it is probably not as efficient as cocontractions of the transverse abdominus and multifidus muscles [58]. This hypothesis was generated by investigating the intra-abdominal pressure change associated with each contraction type [65]. Regardless, cocontractions that recruit abdominal muscles may generate intra-abdominal pressure to stabilize the lumbar segments during most movements [66–68].

LOW BACK PAIN, CORE STABILITY, AND EXERCISE

Persons who have LBP tend to have weakness and imbalances in the muscles that surround the hips and pelvis [36–38] which may absorb impact forces of running and walking less efficiently. The failure to absorb the forces of gait with weak lower extremity muscles may impose high demand on lumbar spine-stabilizing muscles during gait and exercise [36]. It is concerning that people who have LBP exhibit increased lumbar paraspinal muscle activity during gait [69] and lifting exertions [70]. Higher demand placed on weaker, fatigable, unbalanced, and possibly inhibited muscles may prevent patients from being active or result in harmful neuromuscular or postural adaptations during exercise. During prolonged exercise, neuromuscular adaptations in people who have LBP may alter gait mechanics placing lower extremity joints, including the sacral and lumbar spine, at risk for injury or degeneration.

Patients who have LBP commonly exhibit fear of pain or reinjury because of movement [71,72] possibly resulting in gait adaptations including slower walking speeds [67]. Accordingly, LBP sufferers perceive they are less physically active compared with their preinjury condition [8] and may continue to perceive pain and disability related to back pain a year after onset despite the lack of physician consultation after 3 months [73]. This is of concern for LBP sufferers who want, or need, to maintain an active lifestyle. LBP sufferers may adapt to their pain and disability through coping mechanisms to continue their normal activities possibly through self-treating/medicating or through modification/limitation of activities. Formal patient education and guided exercise intervention can reduce frequency of LBP recurrence and severity of individual episodes of LBP [74] and help chronic LBP sufferers to return to work or normal activities [75–77].

There is an abundance of information in the medical literature about kinematic variables and specific temporal patterns of gait in people who have LBP, including stride length, cadence and speed. People who have LBP tend to walk at slower speeds [68,78] and tend to take shorter strides during gait [79]. Kinematic differences during activity in people who have LBP exist, including differences in hip range of motion and increased stride–stride variability [78,80]. People who have LBP also may exhibit lateral trunk list (deviation of the trunk over the pelvis) [79] and reduced lumbar lordosis [41] that likely will cause a more anterior position of the trunk. Changes in trunk positioning during standing or during gait is of concern for people who have LBP because of the possibility of altered spatial location of the body's center of gravity, which may result in a reorganization of lower extremity movements and forces during gait. For example, LBP sufferers walk with reduced hip extension range of motion [81] and may use different adaptive mechanisms while walking at more challenging, faster speeds [69], including increased lumbar muscle activity [82,83]. This increase in lumbar paraspinal muscle activity may be an adaptive mechanism for more efficient center of gravity location and avoid anterior and/or lateral deviations of the trunk.

Surface electromyography has been used to measure paraspinal muscle endurance during lumbar extension exercise as a shift in the median frequency (MedF) of the EMG power spectrum [84]. MedF shifts provide an "appropriate representation of biochemical events" during sustained, fatiguing contractions and describe a change in recruitment from high frequency to low frequency motor units [85]. High fatigability (quicker rates of MedF shift during fatiguing exercise) of the lumbar paraspinal muscles is associated with the presence of and risk for developing LBP [85]. Therefore it is likely that people who have a history of LBP will exhibit different rates of fatigue in the paraspinal muscles during prolonged exercise. Because the force producing capacity of a muscle is reduced as it fatigues, people who have LBP may require a compensatory strategy from surrounding muscles to maintain the desired level of activity or function.

MODELS OF CORE INSTABILITY

Poor lumbar extension endurance, measured as the duration of sustained isometric contraction of the lumbar paraspinals (ie, the Biering-Sorensen test), has been identified as a risk factor for developing LBP [86–88]. Likewise, people who have current LBP [89] or a history of LBP [90] exhibit poor lumbar extension endurance compared with controls. Therefore, people who have poor lumbar spinal endurance may progress quickly to a state of core instability during exercise. These models may contribute to the understanding of the recurrent nature of LBP. Research using isolated lumbar paraspinal fatigue [91] creates a simulated condition of poor core stability to study potential adaptations during exercise in controlled settings.

In healthy individuals, localized lumbar paraspinal fatigue caused deteriorated standing postural control [92] and produced a forward-leaned position of the body, defined as an anterior excursion of the center of pressure and center of mass during static stance [91,92]. In addition, the variability in anterior–posterior and medial–lateral trunk displacement following lumbar paraspinal fatigue was increased significantly during static stance [92]. This finding supports previous findings that lumbar paraspinal fatigue causes deteriorated trunk proprioception [93], which also has been observed in persons with chronic low back pain [94]. These neuromuscular changes suggest that fatigue in muscles that stabilize the core is accompanied by a coping mechanism that may increase risk for falls, thereby increasing the risk for injury and reducing quality of life. In people who have recurrent LBP and core instability, the lumbar spine musculature is likely to fatigue quicker, relative to surrounding muscles, during exercise or activity. Therefore, the body may adapt, through positional and neuromuscular changes during gait, to maintain symmetry and balance while preserving function.

There are also neuromuscular adaptations in response to local lumbar paraspinal fatigue. Immediately following lumbar paraspinal fatigue, healthy subjects experienced a reduction in quadriceps neural activation (measured with the superimposed burst technique) [21,22,24], suggesting a reduced ability to voluntarily recruit quadriceps motor units, despite the fact that subjects did not experience quadriceps fatigue, and had healthy lower extremity joints. In addition, during jogging gait, healthy people experienced reduced knee joint torques during the loading phase of jogging gait immediately following lumbar paraspinal fatigue [24]. Reduced knee joint torques, suggesting a quadriceps avoidance strategy, has been observed in people who have knee joint injury or degeneration. A similar pattern, however, was observed in healthy people without knee injury. Finally, fatigue in the hamstring muscles explained variance in increased quadriceps inhibition following fatiguing isometric lumbar extension exercise in people who had recurrent LBP, not controls [23]. This suggests that people who have LBP may be using their hamstring muscles more as an adaptive mechanism following lumbar fatigue, possibly because of existing weakness in those muscles.

CORE INSTABILITY AND LOWER EXTREMITY INJURY RISK

The relationship between the lumbar/pelvic and hip regions with the remainder of the lower extremity is intuitive. Clinicians routinely evaluate knee, leg, ankle, and foot mechanics in people who have LBP. Likewise, it is common to evaluate for pelvic obliquities in the presence of lower extremity overuse syndromes and other injuries. In a recent review article, Wilson and colleagues [47] wrote, "core stability may provide several benefits to the musculoskeletal system, from maintaining low back health to preventing knee injury." This statement is supported by recent knee injury epidemiologic studies suggesting that lower extremity injury risk may be explained partially by neuromuscular function of the core. Zazulak and colleagues [95] measured transverse plane trunk proprioception in athletes and followed them prospectively for 3 years. They reported a mean, statistically significant difference of 0.7° in transverse plane trunk active reposition error in females who experienced knee joint injuries compared with females who did not sustain knee injury during the follow-up period. This small difference resulted in an 2.9-fold increased odds ratio for experiencing a knee injury for every degree in increased transverse plane active position error. In addition, small differences in maximum flexion, extension, and lateral trunk displacement in response to a sudden perturbation was a significant predictor for knee ligament injury, with 91% sensitivity and 68% specificity, indicating that greater trunk displacements predict knee ligament injury [96]. Therefore, small differences in core proprioception and neuromuscular control may have profound effects on lower extremity injury risk in active populations.

Changes in posture in the presence of core instability may exist during exercise. It has been proposed that people who have chronic LBP exhibit more forward-leaned postures, which may be because of the loss of lumbar lordosis commonly seen in people who have LBP. In theory, a forward-leaned posture or a reduction in trunk proprioception would cause a shift the center of mass, resulting in a reorganization of lower extremity moments during activity. For example, in the sagittal plane, a more anteriorly displaced center of mass would cause ground reaction forces to pass closer to the knee joint in the sagittal plane, resulting in altered knee joint mechanics. This is concerning since poor ground reaction force attenuation by eccentric quadriceps activity may lead to proximal transmission of forces through the knee, hip, and lumbar spine joints. This combined with the possibility of reduced quadriceps muscle activation (increased inhibition) in the presence of lumbar paraspinal fatigue leaving the musculature of the lumbar spine responsible to absorb an excessive amount of force. In the presence of core instability, the muscles surrounding the spine may be fatigued and/or unconditioned and unable to efficiently provide stability. In essence, this creates an environment for the lumbar spine where excessive demand is placed on weak and inhibited muscles, placing the surrounding static stabilizing tissues of the lumbar spine, pelvis, and hips at risk for injury or degenerative processes. This cycle of neuromuscular, kinetic, and kinematic events may explain the recurrent nature of nonspecific low back pain in the active individual and is an area of future investigation involving models of core instability and exercise models with people who have LBP.

SUMMARY

Recurrent and nonspecific LBP presents a clinical dilemma for the treating clinician, because it is a major source of pain, limited activity levels, and reduced quality of life in patients. Weakness, imbalance, poor endurance, and motor control in the muscles that stabilize the core are a likely culprit that can be addressed easily with a multidisciplinary strategy including rehabilitation and exercise prescription. Neuromuscular and postural adaptations occurring as a result of poor core stability may explain the recurrent nature of low back pain and may place lower extremity joints at risk for injury or degenerative processes.

References

[1] Lawrence JP, Greene HS, Grauer JN. Back pain in athletes. J Am Acad Orthop Surg 2006;14(13):726–35.
[2] Papageorgiou AC, Croft PR, Ferry S, et al. Estimating the prevalence of low back pain in the general population. Evidence from the South Manchester Back Pain Survey. Spine 1995; 20(17):1889–94.
[3] Andersson G. The epidemiology of spinal disorders. In: Frymoyer J, editor. The adult spine. New York: Raven Press; 1997. p. 93–141.
[4] Andersson GB. Epidemiological features of chronic low back pain. Lancet 1999;354(9178):581–5.
[5] Frymoyer JW, Cats-Baril WL. An overview of the incidences and costs of low back pain. Orthop Clin North Am 1991;22(2):263–71.
[6] Coste J, Spira A, Ducimetiere P, et al. Clinical and psychological diversity of nonspecific low back pain. A new approach towards the classification of clinical subgroups. J Clin Epidemiol 1991;44(11):1233–45.
[7] Ozguler A, Leclerc A, Landre MF, et al. Individual and occupational determinants of low back pain according to various definitions of low back pain. J Epidemiol Community Health 2000;54(3):215–20.
[8] Verbunt JA, Sieben JM, Seelen HA, et al. Decline in physical activity, disability, and pain-related fear in subacute low back pain. Eur J Pain 2005;9(4):417–25.
[9] MacDonald MJ, Sorock GS, Volinn E, et al. A descriptive study of recurrent low back pain claims. J Occup Environ Med 1997;39(1):35–43.
[10] Keller A, Hayden J, Bombardier C, et al. Effect sizes of nonsurgical treatments of nonspecific low back pain. Eur Spine J 2007;16(11):1776–88.
[11] Fairbank JC, Pynsent PB. The Oswestry Disability Index. Spine 2000;25(22):2940–52 [discussion: 2952].
[12] Meade T, Browne W, Mellows S, et al. Comparison of chiropractic and hospital outpatient management of low back pain: a feasibility study. J Epidemiol Community Health 1986;40: 12–7.
[13] Fairbank JC. The use of revised Oswestry Disability Questionnaire. Spine 2000;25(21): 2846–7.

[14] Gronblad M, Hupli M, Wennerstrand P, et al. Intercorrelation and test–retest reliability of the Pain Disability Index (PDI) and the Oswestry Disability Questionnaire (ODQ) and their correlation with pain intensity in low back pain patients. Clin J Pain 1993;9(3): 189–95.

[15] Fairbank JC, Couper J, Davies JB, et al. The Oswestry Low Back Pain Disability Questionnaire. Physiotherapy 1980;66(8):271–3.

[16] Roland M, Morris R. A study of the natural history of back pain. Part I: development of a reliable and sensitive measure of disability in low back pain. Spine 1983;8(2):141–4.

[17] Roland M, Morris R. A study of the natural history of low back pain. Part II: development of guidelines for trials of treatment in primary care. Spine 1983;8(2):145–50.

[18] Jensen MP, Strom SE, Turner JA, et al. Validity of the Sickness Impact Profile Roland scale as a measure of dysfunction in chronic pain patients. Pain 1992;50(2):157–62.

[19] Beurskens AJ, de Vet HC, Koke AJ. Responsiveness of functional status in low back pain: a comparison of different instruments. Pain 1996;65(1):71–6.

[20] Roland M, Fairbank J. The Roland-Morris Disability Questionnaire and the Oswestry Disability Questionnaire. Spine 2000;25(24):3115–24.

[21] Hart JM, Fritz JM, Kerrigan DC, et al. Reduced quadriceps activation after lumbar paraspinal fatiguing exercise. J Athl Train 2006;41(1):79–86.

[22] Hart JM, Fritz JM, Kerrigan DC, et al. Quadriceps inhibition after repetitive lumbar extension exercise in persons with a history of low back pain. J Athl Train 2006;41(3):264–9.

[23] Hart JM, Kerrigan DC, Fritz JM, et al. Contribution of hamstring fatigue to quadriceps inhibition following lumbar extension exercise. Journal of Sports Science and Medicine 2006;2006(5):70–9.

[24] Hart JM. Quadriceps inhibition and gait kinetics following fatiguing isometric lumbar paraspinal exercise [dissertation]. Charlottesville (VA): Sports Medicine/Athletic Training, University of Virginia; 2005.

[25] Bogduk N. The anatomical basis for spinal pain syndromes. J Manipulative Physiol Ther 1995;18(9):603–5.

[26] Dreyer SJ, Dreyfuss PH. Low back pain and the zygapophysial (facet) joints. Arch Phys Med Rehabil 1996;77(3):290–300.

[27] Schwarzer AC, Aprill CN, Derby R, et al. The relative contributions of the disc and zygapophyseal joint in chronic low back pain. Spine 1994;19(7):801–6.

[28] Maigne JY, Lagauche D, Doursounian L. Instability of the coccyx in coccydynia. J Bone Joint Surg Br 2000;82(7):1038–41.

[29] Kent PM, Keating JL. The epidemiology of low back pain in primary care. Chiropr Osteopat 2005;13:13.

[30] Trainor TJ, Wiesel SW. Epidemiology of back pain in the athlete. Clin Sports Med 2002;21(1):93–103.

[31] Trainor TJ, Trainor MA. Etiology of low back pain in athletes. Curr Sports Med Rep 2004;3(1):41–6.

[32] Bono CM. Low back pain in athletes. J Bone Joint Surg Am 2004;86-A(2):382–96.

[33] Waddell G. Low back pain: a twentieth century health care enigma. Spine 1996;21(24): 2820–5.

[34] Biering-Sorensen F. A prospective study of low back pain in a general population. I. Occurrence, recurrence, and aetiology. Scand J Rehabil Med 1983;15(2):71–9.

[35] Wasiak R, Pransky G, Verma S, et al. Recurrence of low back pain: definition–sensitivity analysis using administrative data. Spine 2003;28(19):2283–91.

[36] Nadler SF, Malanga GA, DePrince M, et al. The relationship between lower extremity injury, low back pain, and hip muscle strength in male and female collegiate athletes. Clin J Sport Med 2000;10(2):89–97.

[37] Nadler SF, Malanga GA, Feinberg JH, et al. Relationship between hip muscle imbalance and occurrence of low back pain in collegiate athletes: a prospective study. Am J Phys Med Rehabil 2001;80(8):572–7.

[38] Nadler SF, Malanga GA, Bartoli LA, et al. Hip muscle imbalance and low back pain in athletes: influence of core strengthening. Med Sci Sports Exerc 2002;34(1):9–16.

[39] Jones MA, Stratton G, Reilly T, et al. Biological risk indicators for recurrent nonspecific low back pain in adolescents. Br J Sports Med 2005;39(3):137–40.

[40] McClure PW, Esola M, Schreier R, et al. Kinematic analysis of lumbar and hip motion while rising from a forward, flexed position in patients with and without a history of low back pain. Spine 1997;22(5):552–8.

[41] Hultman G, Saraste H, Ohlsen H. Anthropometry, spinal canal width, and flexibility of the spine and hamstring muscles in 45–55-year-old men with and without low back pain. J Spinal Disord 1992;5(3):245–53.

[42] Panjabi MM. Clinical spinal instability and low back pain. J Electromyogr Kinesiol 2003;13(4):371–9.

[43] Panjabi MM. The stabilizing system of the spine. Part II. Neutral zone and instability hypothesis. J Spinal Disord 1992;5(4):390–6 [discussion: 397].

[44] Panjabi MM. The stabilizing system of the spine. Part I. Function, dysfunction, adaptation, and enhancement. J Spinal Disord 1992;5(4):383–9 [discussion: 397].

[45] Comerford MJ, Mottram SL. Movement and stability dysfunction—contemporary developments. Man Ther 2001;6(1):15–26.

[46] Comerford MJ, Mottram SL. Functional stability retraining: principles and strategies for managing mechanical dysfunction. Man Ther 2001;6(1):3–14.

[47] Willson JD, Dougherty CP, Ireland ML, et al. Core stability and its relationship to lower extremity function and injury. J Am Acad Orthop Surg 2005;13(5):316–25.

[48] Leetun DT, Ireland ML, Willson JD, et al. Core stability measures as risk factors for lower extremity injury in athletes. Med Sci Sports Exerc 2004;36(6):926–34.

[49] Kibler WB, Press J, Sciascia A. The role of core stability in athletic function. Sports Med 2006;36(3):189–98.

[50] Bergmark A. Stability of the lumbar spine. A study in mechanical engineering. Acta Orthop Scand Suppl 1989;230:1–54.

[51] Hodges PW. Changes in motor planning of feedforward postural responses of the trunk muscles in low back pain. Exp Brain Res 2001;141(2):261–6.

[52] Hodges PW, Richardson CA. Delayed postural contraction of transversus abdominis in low back pain associated with movement of the lower limb. J Spinal Disord 1998;11(1):46–56.

[53] Hodges PW, Richardson CA. Altered trunk muscle recruitment in people with low back pain with upper limb movement at different speeds. Arch Phys Med Rehabil 1999;80(9):1005–12.

[54] Panjabi MM. Lumbar spine instability: a biomechanical challenge. Curr Orthop 1994;8(2):100–5.

[55] Cholewicki J, McGill SM. Lumbar posterior ligament involvement during extremely heavy lifts estimated from fluoroscopic measurements. J Biomech 1992;25(1):17–28.

[56] Panjabi M, Abumi K, Duranceau J, et al. Spinal stability and intersegmental muscle forces. A biomechanical model. Spine 1989;14(2):194–200.

[57] Hodges PW, Richardson CA. Contraction of the abdominal muscles associated with movement of the lower limb. Phys Ther 1997;77(2):132–42 [discussion: 142–14].

[58] Cholewicki J, Juluru K, McGill SM. Intra-abdominal pressure mechanism for stabilizing the lumbar spine. J Biomech 1999;32(1):13–7.

[59] Richardson CA, Jull GA. Muscle control–pain control. What exercises would you prescribe? Man Ther 1995;1(1):2–10.

[60] Richardson CA, Snijders CJ, Hides JA, et al. The relation between the transversus abdominis muscles, sacroiliac joint mechanics, and low back pain. Spine 2002;27(4):399–405.

[61] Richardson C, Jull G, Hodges P, et al. Therapeutic exercise for spinal segmental stabilization in low back pain. London: Churchill Livingstone; 1999.

[62] Sahrmann S. Diagnosis and treatment of movement impairment syndromes. St. Louis (MO): Mosby, Inc.; 2002.

[63] Kennedy B. A muscle-bracing technique utilizing intra-abdominal pressure to stabilize the lumbar spine. Aust J Physiother 1965;11(3):102–6.

[64] van Wingerden JP, Vleeming A, Buyruk HM, et al. Stabilization of the sacroiliac joint in vivo: verification of muscular contribution to force closure of the pelvis. Eur Spine J 2004;13(3): 199–205.

[65] Essendrop M, Schibye B, Hye-Knudsen C. Intra-abdominal pressure increases during exhausting back extension in humans. Eur J Appl Physiol 2002;87(2):167–73.

[66] Lamoth CJ, Meijer OG, Daffertshofer A, et al. Effects of chronic low back pain on trunk coordination and back muscle activity during walking: changes in motor control. Eur Spine J 2006;15(1):23–40.

[67] Al-Obaidi SM, Al-Zoabi B, Al-Shuwaie N, et al. The influence of pain and pain-related fear and disability beliefs on walking velocity in chronic low back pain. Int J Rehabil Res 2003;26(2):101–8.

[68] Khodadadeh S, Eisenstein SM. Gait analysis of patients with low back pain before and after surgery. Spine 1993;18(11):1451–5.

[69] Arendt-Nielsen L, Graven-Nielsen T, Svarrer H, et al. The influence of low back pain on muscle activity and coordination during gait: a clinical and experimental study. Pain 1996;64(2):231–40.

[70] Ferguson SA, Marras WS, Burr DL, et al. Differences in motor recruitment and resulting kinematics between low back pain patients and asymptomatic participants during lifting exertions. Clin Biomech (Bristol, Avon) 2004;19(10):992–9.

[71] Sieben JM, Vlaeyen JW, Tuerlinckx S, et al. Pain-related fear in acute low back pain: the first two weeks of a new episode. Eur J Pain 2002;6(3):229–37.

[72] Sieben JM, Portegijs PJ, Vlaeyen JW, et al. Pain-related fear at the start of a new low back pain episode. Eur J Pain 2005;9(6):635–41.

[73] Croft PR, Macfarlane GJ, Papageorgiou AC, et al. Outcome of low back pain in general practice: a prospective study. BMJ 1998;316(7141):1356–9.

[74] Lonn JH, Glomsrod B, Soukup MG, et al. Active back school: prophylactic management for low back pain. A randomized, controlled, 1-year follow-up study. Spine 1999;24(9): 865–71.

[75] van Tulder MW, Malmivaara A, Esmail R, et al. Exercise therapy for low back pain. Cochrane Database Syst Rev 2000;(2):CD000335.

[76] Casazza BA, Young JL, Herring SA. The role of exercise in the prevention and management of acute low back pain. Occup Med 1998;13(1):47–60.

[77] van Tulder MW, Koes BW, Bouter LM. Conservative treatment of acute and chronic nonspecific low back pain. A systematic review of randomized controlled trials of the most common interventions. Spine 1997;22(18):2128–56.

[78] Vogt L, Pfeifer K, Portscher M, et al. Influences of nonspecific low back pain on three-dimensional lumbar spine kinematics in locomotion. Spine 2001;26(17):1910–9.

[79] Gillan MG, Ross JC, McLean IP, et al. The natural history of trunk list, its associated disability, and the influence of McKenzie management. Eur Spine J 1998;7(6):480–3.

[80] Vogt L, Pfeifer K, Banzer W. Neuromuscular control of walking with chronic low back pain. Man Ther 2003;8(1):21–8.

[81] Lamoth CJ, Daffertshofer A, Meijer OG, et al. How do persons with chronic low back pain speed up and slow down? Trunk–pelvis coordination and lumbar erector spinae activity during gait. Gait Posture 2006;23(2):230–9.

[82] Dedering A, Nemeth G, Harms-Ringdahl K. Correlation between electromyographic spectral changes and subjective assessment of lumbar muscle fatigue in subjects without pain from the lower back. Clin Biomech (Bristol, Avon) 1999;14(2):103–11.

[83] Kramer M, Ebert V, Kinzl L, et al. Surface electromyography of the paravertebral muscles in patients with chronic low back pain. Arch Phys Med Rehabil 2005;86(1):31–6.

[84] Basmajian JV, De Luca CJ. Muscles alive: their functions revealed by electromyography. Baltimore (MD): Williams & Wilkins; 1985.

[85] Mannion AF, Connolly B, Wood K, et al. The use of surface EMG power spectral analysis in the evaluation of back muscle function. J Rehabil Res Dev 1997;34(4):427–39.

[86] Biering-Sorensen F. Physical measurements as risk indicators for low-back trouble over a one-year period. Spine 1984;9(2):106–19.

[87] Biering-Sorensen F. A one-year prospective study of low back trouble in a general population. The prognostic value of low back history and physical measurements. Dan Med Bull 1984;31(5):362–75.

[88] Biering-Sorensen F, Thomsen CE, Hilden J. Risk indicators for low back trouble. Scand J Rehabil Med 1989;21(3):151–7.

[89] Latimer J, Maher CG, Refshauge K, et al. The reliability and validity of the Biering-Sorensen test in asymptomatic subjects and subjects reporting current or previous nonspecific low back pain. Spine 1999;24(20):2085–9 [discussion 2090].

[90] Simmonds MJ, Olson SL, Jones S, et al. Psychometric characteristics and clinical usefulness of physical performance tests in patients with low back pain. Spine 1998;23(22): 2412–21.

[91] Davidson BS, Madigan ML, Nussbaum MA. Effects of lumbar extensor fatigue and fatigue rate on postural sway. Eur J Appl Physiol 2004;93(1-2):183–9.

[92] Madigan ML, Davidson BS, Nussbaum MA. Postural sway and joint kinematics during quiet standing are affected by lumbar extensor fatigue. Hum Mov Sci 2006;25(6):788–99.

[93] Taimela S, Kankaanpaa M, Luoto S. The effect of lumbar fatigue on the ability to sense a change in lumbar position. A controlled study. Spine 1999;24(13):1322–7.

[94] O'Sullivan P, Mitchell BT, Bulich P, et al. The relationship between posture and back muscle endurance in industrial workers with flexion-related low back pain. Man Ther 2006;11(4): 264–71.

[95] Zazulak BT, Hewett TE, Reeves NP, et al. The effects of core proprioception on knee injury: a prospective biomechanical-epidemiological study. Am J Sports Med 2007;35(3): 368–73.

[96] Zazulak BT, Hewett TE, Reeves NP, et al. Deficits in Neuromuscular Control of the Trunk Predict Knee Injury Risk: A Prospective Biomechanical-Epidemiologic Study. Am J Sports Med 2007;35(7):1123–30.

Clin Sports Med 27 (2008) 463–479

CLINICS IN SPORTS MEDICINE

ELSEVIER
SAUNDERS

Clinical Prediction for Success of Interventions for Managing Low Back Pain

Jeffrey Hebert, DC[a],*, Shane Koppenhaver, MPT[a],
Julie Fritz, PhD, PT, ATC[a], Eric Parent, PhD, PT[b]

[a]The University of Utah, College of Health, 520 Wakara Way, Salt Lake City, UT 84108, USA
[b]Department of Physical Therapy, The University of Alberta, Faculty of Rehabilitation Medicine, Edmonton, Canada

L
ow back pain (LBP) is highly prevalent in athletic and nonathletic populations, and is a common cause of pain and disability. It is difficult to identify the pathoanatomical cause for most cases of LBP, leading many to consider LBP as a single "nonspecific" disorder. Most studies evaluating the treatment effectiveness of interventions for LBP have been based on this presumption and have generally demonstrated small to no treatment effects. Most providers think of LBP as a more heterogeneous disorder, and the inability to more specifically match patients to interventions likely to be beneficial is one possible explanation for the lack of research evidence proving the effectiveness of treatments and the suboptimal outcomes of clinical care. Treatment-based classification, one approach to subgrouping patients with "nonspecific" LBP, focuses on identifying clusters of findings from the history and clinical examination that predict a more favorable outcome with a specific treatment approach. By matching patients with the appropriate specific exercise, stabilization exercise, spinal manipulation, or traction treatment, providers may expect a high probability of a successful clinical outcome.

LBP imposes an enormous burden in the United States, both to individuals and to society. LBP is the most common type of pain reported by adults [1], and is among the most frequent complaints seen in physicians' offices [2]. Moreover, 60% of LBP sufferers experience some form of functional limitation or disability as a result of their pain [3]. Pain and disability attributable to LBP are accompanied by an estimated $100 billion to $200 billion in health care expenditures and lost wages annually in the United States [4], equivalent to over 1% of the entire gross domestic product. Despite many recent advances in

*Corresponding author. Division of Physical Therapy, 520 Wakara Way, Salt Lake City, UT 84108. E-mail address: jeff.hebert@utah.edu (J. Hebert).

0278-5919/08/$ – see front matter
doi:10.1016/j.csm.2008.03.002
sportsmed.theclinics.com

imaging and surgical technology, LBP prevalence and its related economic and societal burden have remained largely unchanged in the past decade [1,4].

Athletes may be especially susceptible to LBP and low back injuries. The prevalence of LBP appears particularly high for participants in sports that place high demands on the spine, such as wrestling, gymnastics, and golf [5]. Among the general population, LBP symptoms only weakly correlate with abnormal imaging findings and the great majority of cases of LBP cannot be attributed to specific pathoanatomical causes [6]. Athletes may be more likely than non-athletes to have an identifiable pathoanatomical cause of LBP symptoms [7,8]. Higher rates of spondylolysis, spondylolisthesis, and disc degeneration have been reported in athletes than in the general population [9,10]. Despite an increased incidence of certain pathoanatomical findings, it remains difficult to identify a specific cause in the majority of cases of LBP in athletes. The inability to identify a cause can make it difficult for clinicians to determine which treatment strategy is most likely to be effective. To assist clinicians in predicting which intervention is likely to be most effective, this article reviews the evidence for various interventions commonly used in the treatment of LBP.

SUB-GROUPING PATIENTS WITH LOW BACK PAIN

Common treatment alternatives for individuals with LBP, including those involved in athletics, consist of various forms of exercise, stabilization training, manual therapy, traction, and the use of physical modalities. Physical modalities, such as therapeutic ultrasound and electrical muscle stimulation, are widely used in the treatment of LBP [11], but randomized trials, systematic reviews, and practice guidelines have not supported the efficacy of these approaches [12–18]. Therefore, they are not considered as unique treatment strategies.

Exercise, manual therapy, traction, and many other treatments have been the subject of extensive scientific inquiry. Despite research efforts, evidence showing the effectiveness of these treatments is generally lacking or inconclusive. Even in studies that show some benefit for these treatments, the magnitude of the observed effects is often small, and the utility of these treatments remains subject to debate [13,16]. This can leave clinicians in a quandary as to the best treatment approach for a patient with LBP. The unfortunate result of this clinical dilemma is that one therapy can appear as appealing as the next, which may lead to less effective and efficient treatment. An increasing volume of information is available, however, to assist clinicians in predicting which type of treatment may be most likely to benefit an individual patient with LBP. Incorporation of this information into practice may improve clinical decision-making and treatment outcomes. A top priority for LBP research is to identify criteria for various subgroups of patients with LBP [19–21]. The nature of these subgroups and the methods for detecting them have been the subjects of a great deal of recent debate and research activity [22].

One approach to subgrouping patients with LBP has focused on identifying clusters of findings from the clinical examination that predict a more favorable outcome with a specific treatment approach [23]. Several experts in rehabilitation, including McKenzie and others, have advocated this treatment-based approach. This article focuses on treatment-based subgrouping hypotheses originally described by Delitto and colleagues in 1995 [24]. The subgrouping hypotheses proposed are intended for patients who may or may not be involved in athletic activities with acute LBP or an acute exacerbation of LBP causing substantial pain and limitations in daily activities. After screening patients for any signs of serious pathology, information collected during the history and physical examination is used to place a patient into a subgroup. The name of each subgroup describes the fundamental treatment approach believed to offer the best chance for a successful outcome: manipulation, specific exercise (flexion, extension, and lateral shift patterns), stabilization, and traction. The cluster of examination findings and treatment strategies associated with each subgroup is reviewed in the following sections.

TREATMENT SUBGROUPS
Specific Exercise
The specific exercise subgroup emphasizes treatment using repeated end-range movements of the lumbar spine in a specific direction to affect the location and intensity of the patient's pain. This relationship between movement and pain was first emphasized by McKenzie [25]. Examination findings believed to identify patients in this subgroup include the presence of symptoms in the lower extremities, signs of nerve root compression (eg, positive straight-leg raise test; diminished reflex, sensation, or strength). The principle finding related to the specific exercise subgroup is the presence of centralization or a directional preference during the examination. Centralization occurs when a movement or position results in the relief of pain or paresthesia, or causes symptoms to move from a distal/lateral position in the buttocks and/or lower extremity to a more proximal location, closer to the midline of the lumbar spine [26]. Research has demonstrated the prognostic importance of the centralization phenomenon in patients with LBP with or without sciatica [27–33]. For example, Werneke and colleagues [32] examined the prognostic value of 23 demographic, psychosocial, occupational, and physical examination variables in 223 consecutive patients with acute LBP. The absence of centralization in this sample was associated with delayed recovery and the development of chronic LBP and disability. A concept related to centralization is directional preference. Directional preference occurs when a movement in one direction relieves pain or increases range of motion, and is often associated with movement in the opposite direction resulting in a worsening of the patient's signs and symptoms [34].

Advocates of a treatment-based classification approach contend that the presence of centralization or a directional preference is not just a favorable prognostic finding, but is among the predictive variables indicating the need for a specific exercise approach in treatment (Table 1). The basic treatment premise for patients in the specific exercise subgroup is the use of repeated, or sustained, end-range movements in the direction that caused centralization or of the directional preference determined during the examination. The movement

Table 1
Subgroups of patients with low back pain with subgroup criteria and treatment approaches

Subgroup	Subgroup criteria	Treatment approach
Specific exercise: extension	Symptoms distal to the buttock Symptoms centralize with lumbar extension Symptoms peripheralize with lumbar flexion Directional preference for extension	End-range extension exercises Mobilization to promote extension Avoidance of flexion activities
Specific exercise: flexion	Older age (>50 y) Directional preference for flexion Imaging evidence of lumbar spine stenosis	End-range flexion exercises Mobilization or manipulation of the spine and/or lower extremities Exercise to address impairments of strength or flexibility Body weight–supported ambulation
Stabilization	Younger age (<40 y) Average straight-leg raise (>91°) Aberrant movement present Positive prone-instability test	Exercises to strengthen large spinal muscles (erector spinae, oblique abdominals) Exercises to promote contraction of deep spinal muscles (multifidus, transversus abdominus)
Manipulation	No symptoms distal to knee Duration of symptoms <16 d Lumbar hypomobility Fear-Avoidance Beliefs Questionnaire for Work <19 Hip internal rotation range of motion >35°	Manipulation techniques for the lumbo-pelvic region Active lumbar range-of-motion exercises
Traction	Symptoms extend distal to the buttock(s) Signs of nerve root compression Peripheralization with extension movement; or positive contralateral straight-leg raise test	Prone mechanical traction Extension-specific exercises

may be flexion, extension, or lateral translation. The most common specific exercise movement for younger individuals or athletes is extension [35]. Treatments for patients who centralize or demonstrate a preference for extension include repeated end-range extension exercises, such as prone press-ups

(Fig. 1), or lumbar extension performed while standing. Exercises are progressed by increasing the amount of force or increasing the range of motion to maximize symptom relief. It is important that patients in this subgroup perform these activities frequently throughout the day. Patients may also need to be educated to avoid activities that promote prolonged or end-range flexion activities, such as lifting with poor body mechanics or sitting for long periods. Mobilization of the lumbar spine into extension (eg, posterior-to-anterior mobilization) may also be a useful treatment adjunct. An important contraindication to repeated end-range extension activities that should be considered in athletes with LBP is spondylolisthesis.

Several studies have investigated the effectiveness of an extension-specific exercise treatment approach. Studies that have applied this treatment to patients who fit the subgrouping criteria described above have reported evidence favoring the approach over other exercise interventions [36,37]. Trials that have evaluated an extension-specific exercise approach without an attempt to limit patients to those with these subgrouping criteria have generally not supported the effectiveness of this treatment option [38–41]. For example, Long and colleagues [35] randomized 230 patients with LBP who had a directional preference to receive either usual care, specific exercises in the direction of their preference, or specific exercises in the direction opposite their preference. The directional preference was extension for 83% of patients. Patients receiving exercises in the matched direction showed greater reductions in pain and disability after 2 weeks of treatment [35]. Browder and colleagues [35] randomized 48 patients with LBP who centralized with extension to receive either an extension-specific exercise approach or stabilization exercises. Patients receiving the extension-specific exercise approach, which included extension exercises, patient education, and graded posterior-to-anterior mobilization, showed greater improvement in disability at both short- (1- and 4-week), and long-term (6-month) outcomes [35].

Stabilization Exercise

Functional deficits of the trunk muscles have been observed in general [42,43,44] and athletic [45,46] populations with LBP. Similar deficits in trunk

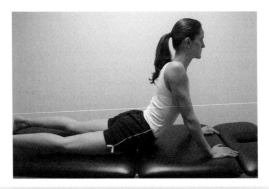

Fig. 1. Example of specific exercise: prone press-up.

muscle function have also been associated with traumatic knee injury [47,48] and chronic groin pain in athletes [49], suggesting that a lack of trunk control may compromise function or stability of the lower extremities during athletic activity. In addition to deficits in neuromuscular control of the trunk muscles, patients with LBP have also been observed to have morphologic changes, including atrophy [50–54] and fatty infiltration [55–57] in the lumbar multifidus and erector spinae muscles. Stabilization exercise programs are typically designed to address the deficits in strength, endurance, and function of the trunk musculature that have been identified in patients with LBP. It is thought that improvements in trunk muscle function lead to decreases in pain and disability by improving the control of spinal segments during movement. In support of this hypothesis, stabilization exercise has been shown to improve trunk muscle function [58,59] and morphology [60–62] in individuals with LBP.

Improvements in trunk muscle function and morphology may represent important outcomes of rehabilitation programs. However, these physiologic changes may not correspond to patient-centered improvements in pain and disability. This concern is highlighted by the conflicting results of research examining the effects of stabilization exercise programs on patient-centered outcomes. While some studies support stabilization exercises as an effective treatment for LBP [63–66], others have demonstrated equivalence between stabilization exercise and traditional rehabilitation approaches [67] or manual therapy [68,69]. A recent systematic review by Rackwitz and colleagues [70] concluded that stabilization exercise for LBP is more effective than treatment by a general practitioner but not more effective than other physiotherapy interventions.

Conflicting findings of research evaluating the effectiveness of stabilization exercise support the consideration that there may be a subgroup of patients with LBP who are most likely to benefit from this approach. Hicks and colleagues [71] investigated variables that may identify which patients with LBP are likely to experience clinical success when receiving stabilization exercises. Four variables (see Table 1) were most predictive of success, defined as a 50% reduction in disability as measured by the Oswestry Questionnaire. When three or more of these variables were present, the probability of achieving clinical success increased from 33% to 67%. While the presence of these variables was associated with an increased likelihood of success, it is clear that future research may be able to identify additional factors to improve the prediction of success with stabilization exercises.

The most effective exercises for use in a stabilization program are also a matter of current debate. A good deal of recent attention and research has focused on specific retraining exercises for the deep trunk muscles, in particular the transversus abdominus and multifidus [58,60,64]. The goal of this approach is to retrain the normal stabilizing motor patterns of these muscles, which are often compromised in individuals with LBP. Some evidence for this approach exists [58,64]. However, most studies have compared this specific retraining approach to management involving no exercise or poorly defined exercise protocols. Other stabilization regimens have placed greater emphasis on exercises designed to improve the strength and endurance of larger, more superficial trunk muscles (ie, erector spinae, oblique abdominals, quadratus lumborum) (Fig. 2) [70,71]. This approach to stabilization exercise emphasizes the use of strengthening exercises that sufficiently challenge these important muscle groups while minimizing potentially harmful compressive and shear loading of the spine. Since the stabilizing activity of any of these muscles is generally that of a low-intensity contraction [72], exercise protocols focus on high repetitions of low-load contractions to promote muscle endurance. Recent research has compared specific muscle retraining programs to this more general stabilization approach [61,63,67]. These studies have not found differences favoring one approach over the other. Although many experts advocate the necessity of specifically retraining the deep spinal muscles, the evidence does not clearly support this perspective. Further research should help define the optimal mix of stabilization exercises for patients with LBP.

Spinal Manipulation

Spinal manipulation is generally defined as the application of a high-velocity, low-amplitude thrust to a joint, which frequently results in an audible "crack" or cavitation [73]. The clinical outcomes associated with spinal manipulation have been the subjects of a great deal of scientific investigation. This research has resulted in several randomized clinical trials [74–77] and systematic reviews [16,78] demonstrating effectiveness for manipulation when compared with placebo or other interventions. However, other trials and reviews have failed to

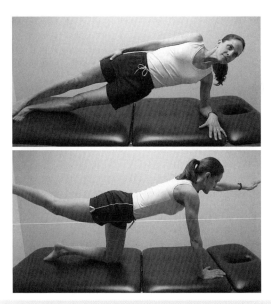

Fig. 2. Examples of stabilization exercises: side bridge (*above*) and bird dog (*below*).

demonstrate a clear clinical benefit of spinal manipulation when compared with other therapies [37,79–81]. Clinical experience suggests that spinal manipulation is effective for at least some patients with LBP. The conflict between research outcomes and clinical experience may be due in part to uncertainty in defining which subgroup of patients with LBP is most likely to benefit from manipulation [82].

Manipulation has been used for centuries [83], yet the mechanism by which manipulation may have a therapeutic effect is subject to debate, which leads to confusion in determining the subgroup that responds best to the treatment. Traditional explanations of the therapeutic mechanism of spinal manipulation have emphasized the importance of directing forces to specific spinal joints for the purpose of correcting a biomechanical dysfunction or misalignment [84–87]. While these constructs may seem intuitive, several studies have questioned their validity. Research has questioned the ability of clinicians to direct manipulative forces in a manner to affect specific spinal joints [88,89]. Furthermore, while there is a small degree of intervertebral movement produced during spinal manipulation [90–92], sustained changes in alignment have not been observed [93].

Flynn and colleagues [94] used a different approach to examining the patient characteristics that may define a subgroup of patients likely to benefit from manipulation by focusing on the prediction of clinical success instead of presumptions based on biomechanical theories. This study identified five variables (see Table 1) predictive of success, defined as a 50% reduction in the Oswestry Questionnaire within 1 week. Patients were considered to be likely responders to manipulation when four or more of these variables were present. When patients met this threshold, the probability of achieving clinical success increased from 45% to 95%.

A follow-up study [76] was performed to examine the validity of these predictive criteria. The results found that patients with LBP receiving manipulation who met these criteria experienced greater decreases in pain and disability than did patients who received manipulation but did not meet the criteria. Additionally, patients who met the criteria and received manipulation experienced greater improvement than did patients who met the criteria but were treated with stabilization exercises. Two important conclusions can be inferred from this study. First, while results do not support spinal manipulation as a superior treatment for all patients with LBP, they do suggest that manipulation is effective for the appropriate subgroup of patients. Second, the presence of these criteria does not automatically equate to a more favorable prognosis unless the appropriate treatment is provided.

The manipulative technique used in this research (Fig. 3) involves a high-velocity, low-amplitude thrust delivered to the anterior superior iliac spine of the supine patient after being sidebent away from and rotated toward the clinician. This procedure was originally thought to be appropriate for patients with biomechanical dysfunction of the sacroiliac articulation [24]. Except for the presence of stiffness somewhere in the lumbar spine, none of the variables

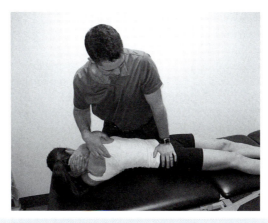

Fig. 3. Manipulation technique.

predictive of success with this procedure related to biomechanical dysfunction. The lack of relationship between clinical success and specific biomechanical dysfunction seems consistent with the growing body of evidence supporting a primarily neurophysiologic mechanism of manipulation. Studies have shown spinal manipulation to affect both sensory and motor nerve activity as well as electromyographic-measured muscle activity [92,95–101]. Although further research is needed, one conclusion can be drawn: If the mechanism of action for spinal manipulation is primarily mediated by neurophysiologic mechanisms rather than biomechanical "realignment," clinicians may be forced to change their paradigm for determining which patients are most appropriate for spinal manipulation.

Traction

Traction techniques for the lumbar spine have a rich history in medicine dating back more than 200 years [102]. Lumbar traction is commonly used [103] and has been referred to by some as "decompression therapy" [104]. Many clinicians believe traction is effective [103,105,106], but the usefulness of traction for treating LBP has been the subject of debate and controversy [107,108].

The traditional presumption of clinicians has considered the presence of sciatica or signs of nerve root compression as indications for traction [103]. Yet, until recently, little research evidence has been available to assist clinicians in predicting which patients with LBP were most likely to benefit from traction. We recently examined the outcomes of patients with LBP who also had symptoms below the buttock and signs of nerve root compression. Our purpose was to determine if these criteria were specific enough to define the subgroup of patients who respond to traction, or if additional criteria were required [27]. We found that the presence of symptoms below the buttock and signs of nerve root compression were not specific enough to define this subgroup of patients. Two additional factors were found to identify patients likely to respond favorably to traction: (1) peripheralization with extension movement and (2) a positive crossed (ie, contralateral) straight-leg raise test. The presence of either of these, in addition to symptoms below the buttock and signs of nerve root compression, define the subgroup of patients who respond to traction. Peripheralization occurs when a movement or posture causes symptoms to move distally, away from the spinal midline. A positive crossed straight-leg raise test is defined as reproduction of the patient's familiar lower extremity symptoms when the contralateral leg is passively raised with the knee maintained in an extended position [109]. When patients with symptoms below the buttock and signs of nerve root compression had either of these findings and received traction along with an extension-specific exercise program, they showed greater short-term reductions in disability than patients with these findings who received only the extension exercise program. These results suggest that traction may be essential to maximize improvement in a specific subgroup of patients (see Table 1).

There has been considerable diversity in the recommended parameters to be used when applying traction. The most common patient position used with mechanical traction is reported to be supine with the hips and knees flexed approximately 90° [103,110]. Although this position is comfortable for many patients with LBP, the position places the lumbar spine in flexion and may therefore be contraindicated for patients who meet the traction subgroup criteria. Pronelying (Fig. 4) may therefore be a preferred position for these patients. There is no clear evidence regarding the most effective traction force. Many experts contend that the force needs to be higher than is typically used in clinical practice (~50% of body weight) to produce a therapeutic effect [111,112]. It may be appropriate to initiate treatment at a slightly lower force (~40% of body weight), then increase the force as tolerated up to a maximum of 60% of body weight. With high-force traction, the duration of treatment may need

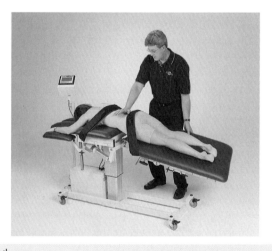

Fig. 4. Traction therapy.

to be shorter (8–12 minutes), with allowances for ramping up and ramping down the force. Because the goal of traction is vertebral separation, static traction is often recommended [111,112]. Traction is rarely delivered as a stand-alone treatment. Because the overall goals of treatment for patients in this subgroup are to reduce and centralize leg symptoms, traction is frequently delivered along with an extension-specific exercise program as described.

Evidence-based guidelines and systematic reviews have not supported the effectiveness of traction for patients with LBP [16,113,114]. The discrepancy between clinical perceptions and research evidence may be attributable to the manner in which traction has been applied in the majority of studies that have examined its effectiveness. Studies that have shown no benefit from using traction have used nonspecific inclusion criteria, essentially allowing all patients fitting a broad definition of acute or chronic LBP to enter [115,116]. Most studies have also failed to adequately define the parameters used for delivering the traction, or have used parameters that are not consistent with expert opinions or typical clinical use [108]. To use traction most effectively, greater attention is needed in the identification of clinical factors that pinpoint patients who need traction and in the application of appropriate dosages of traction.

SUMMARY

The identification of predictive factors in patients with LBP should allow the patient to be matched with the most appropriate treatment intervention, maximizing the likelihood of a favorable clinical outcome [117]. While the identification of predictive factors for the treatment of patients with LBP represents a significant advance in patient care, much more information and research are needed. Nevertheless, it appears that using simple baseline evaluation findings can help clinicians more efficiently and effectively select the most appropriate treatment for an individual patient with LBP.

References

[1] Deyo RA, Mirza SK, Martin BI. Back pain prevalence and visit rates: estimates from U.S. national surveys, 2002. Spine 2006;31(23):2724–7.

[2] Hart LG, Deyo RA, Cherkin DC. Physician office visits for low back pain. Frequency, clinical evaluation, and treatment patterns from a U.S. national survey. Spine 1995;20(1):11–9.

[3] Heliovaara M, Sievers K, Impivaara O, et al. Descriptive epidemiology and public health aspects of low back pain. Ann Med 1989;21(5):327–33.

[4] Katz JN. Lumbar disc disorders and low-back pain: socioeconomic factors and consequences. J Bone Joint Surg Am 2006;88(Suppl 2):21–4.

[5] Bono CM. Low-back pain in athletes. J Bone Joint Surg Am 2004;86(2):382–96.

[6] van Tulder MW, Assendelft WJ, Koes BW, et al. Spinal radiographic findings and nonspecific low back pain. A systematic review of observational studies. Spine 1997;22(4): 427–34.

[7] Hardcastle P, Annear P, Foster DH, et al. Spinal abnormalities in young fast bowlers. J Bone Joint Surg Br 1992;74(3):421–5.

[8] Sward L, Hellstrom M, Jacobsson B, et al. Disc degeneration and associated abnormalities of the spine in elite gymnasts. A magnetic resonance imaging study. Spine 1991;16(4): 437–43.

[9] Ong A, Anderson J, Roche J. A pilot study of the prevalence of lumbar disc degeneration in elite athletes with lower back pain at the Sydney 2000 Olympic Games. Br J Sports Med 2003;37(3):263–6.

[10] McCarroll JR, Miller JM, Ritter MA. Lumbar spondylolysis and spondylolisthesis in college football players. A prospective study. Am J Sports Med 1986;14(5):404–6.

[11] Wong RA, Schumann B, Townsend R, et al. A survey of therapeutic ultrasound use by physical therapists who are orthopaedic certified specialists. Phys Ther 2007;87(8):986–94 [discussion: 995–1001].

[12] Khadilkar A, Milne S, Brosseau L, et al. Transcutaneous electrical nerve stimulation for the treatment of chronic low back pain: a systematic review. Spine 2005;30(23):2657–66.

[13] van Tulder MW, Koes B, Malmivaara A. Outcome of non-invasive treatment modalities on back pain: an evidence-based review. Eur Spine J 2006;15(Suppl 1):S64–81.

[14] Khadilkar A, Milne S, Brosseau L, et al. Transcutaneous electrical nerve stimulation (TENS) for chronic low-back pain. Cochrane Database Syst Rev 2005;(3):CD003008.

[15] Hurwitz EL, Morgenstern H, Kominski GF, et al. A randomized trial of chiropractic and medical care for patients with low back pain: eighteen-month follow-up outcomes from the UCLA low back pain study. Spine 2006;31(6):611–21 [discussion: 622].

[16] Chou R, Huffman LH. Nonpharmacologic therapies for acute and chronic low back pain: a review of the evidence for an American Pain Society/American College of Physicians clinical practice guideline. Ann Intern Med 2007;147(7):492–504.

[17] Philadelphia Panel. Philadelphia Panel evidence-based clinical practice guidelines on selected rehabilitation interventions for low back pain. Phys Ther 2001;81(10):1641–74.

[18] Chou R, Qaseem A, Snow V, et al. Diagnosis and treatment of low back pain: a joint clinical practice guideline from the American College of Physicians and the American Pain Society. Ann Intern Med 2007;147(7):478–91.

[19] Borkan JM, Cherkin DC. An agenda for primary care research on low back pain. Spine 1996;21(24):2880–4.

[20] Borkan JM, Koes B, Reis S, et al. A report from the second international forum for primary care research on low back pain: reexamining priorities. Spine 1998;23(18):1992–6.

[21] Henschke N, Maher CG, Refshauge KM, et al. Low back pain research priorities: a survey of primary care practitioners. BMC Fam Pract 2007;8:40.

[22] Billis EV, McCarthy CJ, Oldham JA. Subclassification of low back pain: a cross-country comparison. Eur Spine J 2007;16(7):865–79.

[23] Riddle DL. Classification and low back pain: a review of the literature and critical analysis of selected systems. Phys Ther 1998;78(7):708–37.

[24] Delitto A, Erhard RE, Bowling RW. A treatment-based classification approach to low back syndrome: identifying and staging patients for conservative management. Phys Ther 1995;75: 470–89.

[25] McKenzie RA. The lumbar spine: mechanical diagnosis and therapy. Waikanae (New Zealand): Spinal Publications Limited; 1989.

[26] Fritz JM, Cleland JA, Childs JD. Subgrouping patients with low back pain: evolution of a classification approach to physical therapy. J Orthop Sports Phys Ther 2007;37(6): 290–302.

[27] Fritz JM, Lindsay W, Matheson JW, et al. Is there a subgroup of patients with low back pain likely to benefit from mechanical traction? Results of a randomized clinical trial and subgrouping analysis. Spine 2007;32(26):E793–800.

[28] Berthelot JM, Delecrin J, Maugars Y, et al. Contribution of centralization phenomenon to the diagnosis, prognosis, and treatment of diskogenic low back pain. Joint Bone Spine 2007;74(4):319–23.

[29] George SZ, Bialosky JE, Donald DA. The centralization phenomenon and fear-avoidance beliefs as prognostic factors for acute low back pain: a preliminary investigation involving patients classified for specific exercise. J Orthop Sports Phys Ther 2005;35(9):580–8.

[30] Karas R, McIntosh G, Hall H, et al. The relationship between nonorganic signs and central-ization of symptoms in the prediction of return to work for patients with low back pain. Phys Ther 1997;77:354–60.

[31] Long AL. The centralization phenomenon. Its usefulness as a predictor or outcome in con-servative treatment of chronic law back pain (a pilot study). Spine 1995;20(23):2513–20 [discussion: 2521].

[32] Werneke M, Hart DL. Centralization phenomenon as a prognostic factor for chronic low back pain and disability. Spine 2001;26(7):758–64 [discussion: 765].

[33] Skytte L, May S, Petersen P. Centralization: its prognostic value in patients with referred symptoms and sciatica. Spine 2005;30(11):E293–9.

[34] Kilpikoski S, Airaksinen O, Kankaanpaa M, et al. Interexaminer reliability of low back pain assessment using the McKenzie method. Spine 2002;27:E207–14.

[35] Long AL, Donelson R. Does it matter which exercise? A randomized trial of exercise for low back pain. Spine 2004;29:2593–602.

[36] Browder DA, Childs JD, Cleland JA, et al. Effectiveness of an extension-oriented treatment approach in a subgroup of subjects with low back pain: a randomized clinical trial. Phys Ther Sep 2007;87(12):1608–18.

[37] Machado LA, de Souza MS, Ferreira PH, et al. The McKenzie method for low back pain: a systematic review of the literature with a meta-analysis approach. Spine 2006;31(9): E254–62.

[38] Cherkin DC, Deyo RA, Battie M, et al. A comparison of physical therapy, chiropractic ma-nipulation, and provision of an educational booklet for the treatment of patients with low back pain. N Engl J Med 1998;339(15):1021–9.

[39] Dettori JR, Bullock SH, Sutlive TG, et al. The effects of spinal flexion and extension exercises and their associated postures in patients with acute low back pain. Spine 1995;20(21): 2303–12.

[40] Indahl A, Velund L, Reikeraas O. Good prognosis for low back pain when left untampered. A randomized clinical trial. Spine 1995;20(4):473–7.

[41] Malmivaara A, Hakkinen U, Aro T, et al. The treatment of acute low back pain—bed rest, exercises, or ordinary activity? N Engl J Med 1995;332(6):351–5.

[42] Hodges PW, Richardson CA. Contraction of the abdominal muscles associated with move-ment of the lower limb. Phys Ther 1997;77(2):132–42.

[43] Hodges PW, Richardson CA. Inefficient muscular stabilization of the lumbar spine associ-ated with low back pain. A motor control evaluation of transversus abdominis. Spine 1996;21:2640–50.

[44] Newcomer KL, Laskowski ER, Yu B, et al. Differences in repositioning error among patients with low back pain compared with control subjects. Spine 2000;25(19): 2488–93.

[45] Reeves NP, Cholewicki J, Silfies SP. Muscle activation imbalance and low-back injury in varsity athletes. J Electromyogr Kinesiol 2006;16(3):264–72.

[46] Renkawitz T, Boluki D, Grifka J. The association of low back pain, neuromuscular imbal-ance, and trunk extension strength in athletes. Spine J 2006;6(6):673–83.

[47] Zazulak BT, Hewett TE, Reeves NP, et al. Deficits in neuromuscular control of the trunk pre-dict knee injury risk: a prospective biomechanical-epidemiologic study. Am J Sports Med 2007;35(7):1123–30.

[48] Zazulak BT, Hewett TE, Reeves NP, et al. The effects of core proprioception on knee injury: a prospective biomechanical-epidemiological study. Am J Sports Med 2007;35(3): 368–73.

[49] Cowan SM, Schache AG, Brukner P, et al. Delayed onset of transversus abdominus in long-standing groin pain. Med Sci Sports Exerc 2004;36(12):2040–5.

[50] Barker KL, Shamley DR, Jackson D. Changes in the cross-sectional area of multifidus and psoas in patients with unilateral back pain: the relationship to pain and disability. Spine 2004;29(22):E515–9.

[51] Danneels LA, Vanderstraeten GG, Cambier DC, et al. CT imaging of trunk muscles in chronic low back pain patients and healthy control subjects. Eur Spine J 2000;9(4): 266–72.

[52] Hides JA, Stokes MJ, Saide M, et al. Evidence of lumbar multifidus muscle wasting ipsilateral to symptoms in patients with acute/subacute low back pain. Spine 1994;19(2): 165–72.

[53] Ng JK, Richardson CA, Kippers V, et al. Relationship between muscle fiber composition and functional capacity of back muscles in healthy subjects and patients with back pain. J Orthop Sports Phys Ther 1998;27(6):389–402.

[54] Yoshihara K, Nakayama Y, Fujii N, et al. Atrophy of the multifidus muscle in patients with lumbar disk herniation: histochemical and electromyographic study. Orthopedics 2003;26(5):493–5.

[55] Kang CH, Shin MJ, Kim SM, et al. MRI of paraspinal muscles in lumbar degenerative kyphosis patients and control patients with chronic low back pain. Clin Radiol 2007;62(5):479–86.

[56] Kjaer P, Bendix T, Sorensen JS, et al. Are MRI-defined fat infiltrations in the multifidus muscles associated with low back pain? BMC Med 2007;5:2.

[57] Mengiardi B, Schmid MR, Boos N, et al. Fat content of lumbar paraspinal muscles in patients with chronic low back pain and in asymptomatic volunteers: quantification with MR spectroscopy. Radiology 2006;240(3):786–92.

[58] Tsao H, Hodges PW. Persistence of improvements in postural strategies following motor control training in people with recurrent low back pain. J Electromyogr Kinesiol 2007, in press.

[59] Tsao H, Hodges PW. Immediate changes in feedforward postural adjustments following voluntary motor training. Exp Brain Res 2007;181(4):537–46.

[60] Hides JA, Richardson CA, Jull GA. Multifidus muscle recovery is not automatic after resolution of acute, first-episode low back pain. Spine 1996;21(23):2763–9.

[61] Danneels LA, Vanderstraeten GG, Cambier DC, et al. Effects of three different training modalities on the cross sectional area of the lumbar multifidus muscle in patients with chronic low back pain. Br J Sports Med 2001;35(3):186–91.

[62] Rissanen A, Kalimo H, Alaranta H. Effect of intensive training on the isokinetic strength and structure of lumbar muscles in patients with chronic low back pain. Spine 1995;20(3): 333–40.

[63] Koumantakis GA, Watson PJ, Oldham JA. Trunk muscle stabilization training plus general exercise versus general exercise only: randomized controlled trial of patients with recurrent low back pain. Phys Ther 2005;85(3):209–25.

[64] Koumantakis GA, Watson PJ, Oldham JA. Supplementation of general endurance exercise with stabilisation training versus general exercise only. Physiological and functional outcomes of a randomised controlled trial of patients with recurrent low back pain. Clin Biomech (Bristol, Avon) 2005;20(5):474–82.

[65] Hides JA, Jull GA, Richardson CA. Long-term effects of specific stabilizing exercises for first-episode low back pain. Spine 2001;26(11):E243–8.

[66] O'Sullivan PB, Phyty GD, Twomey LT, et al. Evaluation of specific stabilizing exercise in the treatment of chronic low back pain with radiologic diagnosis of spondylolysis or spondylolisthesis. Spine 1997;22(24):2959–67.

[67] Cairns MC, Foster NE, Wright C. Randomized controlled trial of specific spinal stabilization exercises and conventional physiotherapy for recurrent low back pain. Spine 2006;31(19):E670–81.

[68] Goldby LJ, Moore AP, Doust J, et al. A randomized controlled trial investigating the efficiency of musculoskeletal physiotherapy on chronic low back disorder. Spine 2006;31(10):1083–93.

[69] Rasmussen-Barr E, Nilsson-Wikmar L, Arvidsson I. Stabilizing training compared with manual treatment in sub-acute and chronic low-back pain. Man Ther 2003;8(4):233–41.

[70] Rackwitz B, de Bie R, Limm H, et al. Segmental stabilizing exercises and low back pain. What is the evidence? A systematic review of randomized controlled trials. Clin Rehabil 2006;20(7):553–67.

[71] Hicks GE, Fritz JM, Delitto A, et al. Preliminary development of a clinical prediction rule for determining which patients with low back pain will respond to a stabilization exercise program. Arch Phys Med Rehabil 2005;86(9):1753–62.

[72] McGill SM. Low back exercises: evidence for improving exercise regimens. Phys Ther 1998;78(7):754–65.

[73] Evans DW. Mechanisms and effects of spinal high-velocity, low-amplitude thrust manipulation: previous theories. J Manipulative Physiol Ther 2002;25(4):251–62.

[74] Aure OF, Nilsen JH, Vasseljen O. Manual therapy and exercise therapy in patients with chronic low back pain: a randomized, controlled trial with 1-year follow-up. Spine 2003;28(6):525–31 [discussion: 531–2].

[75] Team UBT. United Kingdom back pain exercise and manipulation (UK BEAM) randomised trial: effectiveness of physical treatments for back pain in primary care. BMJ 2004;329: 1377–85.

[76] Childs JD, Fritz JM, Flynn TW, et al. A clinical prediction rule to identify patients with low back pain most likely to benefit from spinal manipulation: a validation study. Ann Intern Med 2004;141(12):920–8.

[77] Giles LG, Muller R. Chronic spinal pain: a randomized clinical trial comparing medication, acupuncture, and spinal manipulation. Spine 2003;28(14):1490–502.

[78] Assendelft WJ, Koes BW, van der Heijden GJ, et al. The efficacy of chiropractic manipulation for back pain: blinded review of relevant randomized clinical trials. J Manipulative Physiol Ther 1992;15(8):487–94.

[79] Assendelft WJ, Morton SC, Yu EI, et al. Spinal manipulative therapy for low back pain. Cochrane Database Syst Rev 2004;(1):CD000447.

[80] Cherkin DC, Sherman KJ, Deyo RA, et al. A review of the evidence for the effectiveness, safety, and cost of acupuncture, massage therapy, and spinal manipulation for back pain. Ann Intern Med 2003;138(11):898–906.

[81] Hurwitz EL, Morgenstern H, Harber P, et al. A randomized trial of medical care with and without physical therapy and chiropractic care with and without physical modalities for patients with low back pain: 6-month follow-up outcomes from the UCLA low back pain study. Spine 2002;27(20):2193–204.

[82] Bouter LM, van Tulder MW, Koes BW. Methodologic issues in low back pain research in primary care. Spine 1998;23:2014–20.

[83] Curtis P. Spinal manipulation: does it work? Occup Med 1988;3(1):31–44.

[84] Bernard H. The mechanism of anatomical structure in its relation to osteopathy. 1911. J Am Osteopath Assoc 2000;100(7):444–8.

[85] Cyriax JH. Diagnosis of soft tissue lesions. In: Cyriax JH, editor. Textbook of orthopaedic medicine. 6th edition. Baltimore (MD): Williams & Wilkins; 1976. p. 389.

[86] Maitland GD. Vertebral manipulation. 5th edition. Oxford (UK): Butterworth Heinemann; 1986.

[87] Meeker WC, Haldeman S. Chiropractic: a profession at the crossroads of mainstream and alternative medicine. Ann Intern Med 2002;136(3):216–27.

[88] Ross JK, Bereznick DE, McGill SM. Determining cavitation location during lumbar and thoracic spinal manipulation: Is spinal manipulation accurate and specific? Spine 2004;29(13):1452–7.

[89] Bereznick DE, Ross JK, McGill SM. The frictional properties at the thoracic skin-fascia interface: implications in spine manipulation. Clin Biomech (Bristol, Avon) 2002;17(4): 297–303.

[90] Gal J, Herzog W, Kawchuk G, et al. Movements of vertebrae during manipulative thrusts to unembalmed human cadavers. J Manipulative Physiol Ther 1997;20(1): 30–40.

[91] Maigne JY, Guillon F. Highlighting of interverebral movements and variations of intradiskal pressure during lumbar spine manipulation: a feasibility study. J Manipulative Physiol Ther 2000;23:531–5.

[92] Colloca CJ, Keller TS, Gunzburg R. Biomechanical and neurophysiological responses to spinal manipulation in patients with lumbar radiculopathy. J Manipulative Physiol Ther 2004;27(1):1–15.

[93] Tullberg T, Blomberg S, Branth B, et al. Manipulation does not alter the position of the sacroiliac joint. A roentgen stereophotogrammetric analysis. Spine 1998;23(10):1124–8.

[94] Flynn T, Fritz J, Whitman J, et al. A clinical prediction rule for classifying patients with low back pain who demonstrate short-term improvement with spinal manipulation. Spine 2002;27(24):2835–43.

[95] Colloca CJ, Keller TS, Gunzburg R. Neuromechanical characterization of in vivo lumbar spinal manipulation. Part II. Neurophysiological response. J Manipulative Physiol Ther 2003;26(9):579–91.

[96] Dishman JD, Ball KA, Burke J. First prize: central motor excitability changes after spinal manipulation: a transcranial magnetic stimulation study. J Manipulative Physiol Ther 2002;25(1):1–9.

[97] Dishman JD, Cunningham BM, Burke J. Comparison of tibial nerve H-reflex excitability after cervical and lumbar spine manipulation. J Manipulative Physiol Ther 2002;25(5):318–25.

[98] Herzog W, Scheele D, Conway PJ. Electromyographic responses of back and limb muscles associated with spinal manipulative therapy. Spine 1999;24(2):146–52 [discussion: 153].

[99] Suter E, McMorland G, Herzog W, et al. Decrease in quadriceps inhibition after sacroiliac joint manipulation in patients with anterior knee pain. J Manipulative Physiol Ther 1999;22(3):149–53.

[100] Suter E, McMorland G, Herzog W, et al. Conservative lower back treatment reduces inhibition in knee-extensor muscles: a randomized controlled trial. J Manipulative Physiol Ther 2000;23(2):76–80.

[101] Suter E, McMorland G, Herzog W. Short-term effects of spinal manipulation on H-reflex amplitude in healthy and symptomatic subjects. J Manipulative Physiol Ther 2005;28(9):667–72.

[102] Silver J. The history of modern spinal traction with particular reference to neural disorders. Spinal Cord 1997;35(10):710–1.

[103] Harte AA, Gracey JH, Baxter GD. Current use of lumbar traction in the management of low back pain: results of a survey of physiotherapists in the United Kingdom. Arch Phys Med Rehabil 2005;86(6):1164–9.

[104] Daniel DM. Non-surgical spinal decompression therapy: Does the scientific literature support efficacy claims made in the advertising media? Chiropr Osteopat 2007;15:7.

[105] Mikhail C, Korner-Bitensky N, Rossignoi M, et al. Physical therapists' use of interventions with high evidence of effectiveness in the management of a hypothetical typical patient with acute low back pain. Phys Ther 2005;85:1151–67.

[106] Poitras S, Blais R, Swaine B, et al. Management of work-related low back pain: a population-based survey of physical therapists. Phys Ther 2005;85:1168–81.

[107] Clarke JA, van Tulder MW, Blomberg SE, et al. Traction for low-back pain with or without sciatica. Cochrane Database Syst Rev 2007;(2):CD003010.

[108] Harte AA, Baxter GD, Gracey JH. The efficacy of traction for back pain: a systematic review of randomized controlled trials. Arch Phys Med Rehabil 2003;84(10):1542–53.

[109] Kosteljanetz M, Bang F, Schmidt-Olsen S. The clinical significance of straight-leg raising (Lasegue's sign) in the diagnosis of prolapsed lumbar disc. Interobserver variation and correlation with surgical finding. Spine 1988;13(4):393–5.

[110] Harte AA, Baxter GD, Gracey JH. The effectiveness of motorized lumbar traction in the management of LBP with lumbo sacral nerve root involvement: a feasibility study. BMC Musculoskelet Disord 2007;8:118.

[111] Judovich B. Lumbar traction therapy. JAMA 1955;159:549–52.

[112] Saunders HD. Evaluation, treatment and prevention of musculoskeletal disorders, Vol. 1. 4th edition. Chaska (MN): The Saunders Group; 2004.

[113] Clarke J, van Tulder M, Blomberg S, et al. Traction for low back pain with or without sciatica: an updated systematic review within the framework of the Cochrane collaboration. Spine 2006;31:1591–9.

[114] Macario A, Pergolizzi JV. Systematic literature review of spinal decompression via motorized traction for chronic discogenic low back pain. Pain Pract 2006;6:171–8.

[115] Beurskens AJ, De Vet HC, Koke AJ, et al. Efficacy of traction for nonspecific low back pain. 12-week and 6-month results of a randomized clinical trial. Spine 1997;22:2756–62.

[116] Werners R, Pynsent PB, Bulstrode CJK. Randomized trial comparing interferential therapy with motorized lumbar traction and massage in the management of low back pain in a primary care setting. Spine 1999;24:1579–84.

[117] Brennan GP, Fritz JM, Hunter SJ, et al. Identifying subgroups of patients with acute/subacute "nonspecific" low back pain: results of a randomized clinical trial. Spine 2006;31(6):623–31.

Clin Sports Med 27 (2008) 481–490

CLINICS IN SPORTS MEDICINE

Sensorimotor Factors Affecting Outcome Following Shoulder Injury

Joseph B. Myers, PhD, ATC*, Sakiko Oyama, MS, ATC

University of North Carolina at Chapel Hill, Department of Exercise and Sport Science,
201 Fetzer, CB# 8700, Chapel Hill, NC 27599-8700, USA

When the shoulder is subjected to an injurious mechanism, a cascade of effects results. These effects include tissue pathology and the manifestation of pain. Sensorimotor alterations also manifest, most likely as a result of tissue pathology and pain. The combination of the tissue pathology, pain, and sensorimotor alterations all directly affect outcome following injury, and thus need to be addressed by the clinician treating the shoulder injury to fully restore function. This article discusses how the sensorimotor system contributes to shoulder function and how it is altered with shoulder injury, thereby affecting outcome.

SENSORIMOTOR CONTRIBUTION TO SHOULDER FUNCTION

During activities of daily living, performance of occupational duties, and participation in sport and recreation, more range of motion is required at the shoulder than any other joints. The shoulder range of motion that is observed during functional activities results from the compounding motion achieved by the three joints and one articulation of the shoulder complex, with most of the motion coming from the glenohumeral joint and scapulothoracic articulations. For example, during humeral elevation, if scapulothoracic movement is eliminated, maximum humeral elevation decreases by approximately one third [1–5]. During full humeral elevation, approximately 120 degrees of the overall movement occurs at the glenohumeral joint and approximately 60 degrees occurs at scapulothoracic articulation [1,5]. At the same time, movement at the sternoclavicular joint allows the clavicle to elevate 7 to 15 degrees, retract 15 to 30 degrees, and axially rotate by 15 to 33 degrees [6,7].

To provide this high level of mobility, the glenohumeral joint and scapulothoracic articulation have limited osseus stability [8]. The glenohumeral joint compensates for this limited osseous stability by relying on the other mechanical stabilizing mechanisms achieved by the static structures, including negative

*Corresponding author. E-mail address: joemyers@email.unc.edu (J.B. Myers).

0278-5919/08/$ – see front matter
doi:10.1016/j.csm.2008.03.005

intra-articular pressure, the glenoid labrum, tenomuscular structures, and capsuloligamentous restraints. The static mechanical restraints alone are not enough to provide adequate stability. The shoulder complex therefore relies heavily on dynamic action of the musculature that crosses both the glenohumeral and scapulothoracic articulations to maintain stability while still allowing high mobility.

These static and dynamic mechanisms of stability do not happen independently. The static structures (especially capsuloligamentous structures) influence activation of the muscles that cross the shoulder complex, thus providing stability, through stimulation of mechanoreceptors within the sensorimotor system. The sensorimotor system includes the sensory, motor, and central integration/processing components of the central nervous system (CNS) [9]. Mechanoreceptors are sensory neurons present within joint capsules, ligaments, muscles, tendons, fascia, and skin about a joint [10–12]. Mechanoreceptors are mechanically sensitive and transduce mechanical tissue deformation as frequency-modulated neural signals to the CNS through afferent sensory pathways [10]. Vangsness and colleagues [12] reported that neural endings exist in the shoulder's capsuloligamentous structures. The spiral tightening of the capsule that occurs with abduction and external rotation sequentially tightens the capsuloligamentous structures, and is therefore considered to stimulate those mechanoreceptors [13]. Low-threshold, slow-adapting Ruffini afferents were most abundant overall, except in the glenohumeral ligaments where low-threshold, rapid-adapting Pacinian-type afferents outnumber Ruffini afferents [12]. Ruffini afferents are believed to be stimulated only in extremes of motion through tensile force, acting as limit detectors [10]. Like Ruffini receptors, Pacinian corpuscles respond in extremes of motion, but through combination of compressive and tensile mechanisms, rather than stretching alone [10]. No mechanoreceptors were present in the subacromial bursa or glenoid labrum [12].

Sensory information from these mechanoreceptors travels from the shoulder joint through afferent pathways to the CNS where it is processed and integrated with input from the other levels of the nervous system (central processing), eliciting contractile muscle responses vital to coordinated movement patterns and joint stability [9]. This information is termed proprioception and is defined as the afferent information, arising from peripheral areas of the body (including the mechanical and dynamic restraints about the shoulder), that contributes to joint stability, postural control, and motor control [9,14,15]. Proprioception has three submodalities, which include joint position sense, kinesthesia, and sensation of force [14,15]. Joint position sense is the appreciation and interpretation of information concerning one's joint position and orientation in space. Kinesthesia is the ability to appreciate and interpret joint motions [16]. Sensation of force is the ability to appreciate and interpret force applied to or generated within a joint [16].

These submodalities of proprioception are used by the CNS to elicit appropriate neuromuscular control mechanisms important for joint stability and coordinated movement of the shoulder complex. Neuromuscular control is defined as the subconscious activation of the dynamic restraints about the shoulder in preparation and in response to joint motion and loading for the purpose of maintaining joint stability and function [16]. The neuromuscular control mechanisms include coordinated muscle activation during functional tasks, co-activation of the shoulder musculature (force coupling), muscular reflexes, and regulation of muscle tone and stiffness [16,17].

Coordinated muscle activation refers to the muscle activation patterns necessary to properly perform the desired functional task, including the combined effort of concentric contraction by the agonist muscles, eccentric contraction or reflexive inhibition of the antagonist muscles, and activation of synergistic muscles about the shoulder complex. Proper coordination of the muscles that cross the shoulder complex results in fluid, coordinated completion of the desired task while achieving dynamic stability of the joint.

Coactivation of the dynamic restraints at the shoulder joint is vital to shoulder stabilization. The rotator cuff is essential for dynamic stability by centralizing the humeral head within the glenoid fossa, thus preventing excessive humeral translation [18]. For example, contraction of the subscapularis counteracts contraction of the infraspinatus/teres minor, controlling the excessive humeral translation in the frontal plane, while contraction of the deltoid counteracts contraction of the lower rotator cuff muscles (infraspinatus, teres minor, and subscapularis), controlling the excessive humeral translation in the transverse plane [19]. The resultant force exerted by the rotator cuff muscles produces glenohumeral joint compression, which in turn increases congruency of the articulating surfaces [20]. In addition to the synergistic action of glenohumeral musculatures, the common insertion of the rotator cuff tendons within the joint capsule provides an element of dynamic capsular tension. As the cuff muscles simultaneously contract, the forces generated in their tendinous insertion apply tension to the joint capsule [21–23]. The result is increased capsular tension that aids in drawing the humeral head into the glenoid fossa, supplementing joint stability.

Muscle reflexes also play an essential role in dynamic stability of the shoulder. Jerosch and colleagues [24] arthroscopically demonstrated that a reflex arc (ligamento-muscular reflex) exists between the shoulder capsule and the deltoid, trapezius, pectoralis major, and rotator cuff musculature in the human shoulder. Traditionally, the ligamento-muscular reflex research has centered around the alpha motor neuron being the efferent pathway to the muscle. Although these afferent alpha motor neuron reflexes do exist, the gamma motor-muscle spindle system is also a plausible mechanism that mediates shoulder stability by way of reflex. Specifically, gamma motor-muscle spindle system modulates sensitivity of the alpha motor neuron, thus affecting muscle stiffness and ultimately joint stability [25–28]. Joint stiffness is defined as resistance provided by tissue, joint, or limb to a change in shape and position [29]. It provides the first line of defense for joint stability when force is applied to the joint [30–35]. It provides an immediate and substantial response to perturbation and decreases the latency of the reflexive response, thus improving joint stability [36]. The stiffness provided by the muscles about the shoulder plays a substantial role in how effectively external forces imposed on the musculoskeletal system are transmitted to the CNS [37]. Muscle stiffness is strongly influenced by the level of contraction present [38]. As the intensity of muscle contraction increases, so does stiffness [32,39–42]. Mechanoreceptors play a significant role in regulating muscle stiffness. The muscle spindle system contributes to preprogramming muscle stiffness [27]. Ligament mechanoreceptors can also regulate stiffness by heightening muscle spindle sensitivity by way of increased gamma motor neuron excitation, which influences the amount of muscle stiffness and quickening the stiffness achieved from reflexive muscle activation [25–28,43,44].

EFFECTS OF INJURY ON SENSORIMOTOR SYSTEM

When shoulder injury occurs, tissue pathology and pain result. It is hypothesized that sensorimotor alterations also manifest, resulting from the tissue pathology and pain. The combination of the tissue pathology, pain, and sensorimotor alterations all are believed to directly affect shoulder function and ultimately outcome following injury (Fig. 1). Most of the research investigating the affects of injury on sensorimotor system has been targeted toward examining the sensorimotor alteration in patients who have shoulder instability. Effects of rotator cuff diseases, such as impingement and rotator cuff tears, on the sensorimotor system have also been studied.

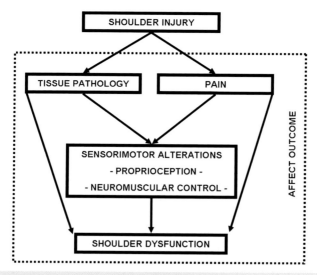

Fig. 1. Effects of shoulder injury on shoulder function.

Sensorimotor Alterations with Shoulder Instability

Sensorimotor alterations have been identified in patients who have various levels of shoulder instability. With traumatic glenohumeral instability, it is believed that the mechanical stimulation of the mechanoreceptors is suppressed because of tissue deafferentation from the trauma or the tissue lengthening (both ligamentous and muscular) [20,45]. Specifically, proprioception deficits, as measured with joint position sense and kinesthesia assessments, have been demonstrated in patients who have shoulder instability [46–48]. A review of the proprioception literature suggests that the tissue lengthening associated with instability is the prime culprit for the sensorimotor deficits. For example, Tibone and colleagues [45] reported that no significant differences in proprioception were present between normal subjects and subjects who had instability, using cortical evoked potential. Given that joint capsule mechanoreceptors were stimulated with electrical potentials rather than from tissue deformation, these results suggest that decreased mechanoreceptor stimulation from capsular laxity, rather than the deafferentation, may be responsible for proprioception deficits in patients who have shoulder instability. In addition, proprioception deficits have been identified in individuals who have atraumatic multidirectional instability [49]. This finding again suggests that the decreased mechanical stimulation rather than tissue deafferentation is the culprit. Patients who have undergone either open or arthroscopic repair to restore capsular tension also demonstrate improved proprioception after surgery [47,48,50–52], suggesting the tissue lengthening and subsequent lack of mechanoreceptor stimulation are associated with the proprioception deficits seen in patients who have instability. Although proprioception is typically improved after surgery, deficits still potentially exist. Fremerey and colleagues [53] demonstrated persisting proprioceptive deficit and an altered EMG pattern following capsulolabral reconstruction. Interestingly, Barden and colleagues [49] demonstrated bilateral deficit in joint position sense in subjects exhibiting unilateral instability. Potzl and colleagues [52] found an improvement in proprioception bilaterally following unilateral surgical intervention. These results suggest that alterations in the central processing mechanisms may also be present.

Neuromuscular control deficits have also been identified in individuals diagnosed with various degrees of instability. Several investigators have assessed the neuromuscular control components of dynamic joint stability in subjects presenting with anterior glenohumeral instability [54–57]. Alterations in coordinated muscle activation pattern were identified in patients who had glenohumeral instability during simple elevation tasks [55,56] and while throwing a baseball [57]. Deficits in coactivation of the rotator cuff and primary humeral movers were present in these patients, possibly leading to compromised dynamic joint stability and further exacerbation of the existing instability [54]. Similarly, Myers and colleagues [54] assessed reflexive characteristics of the shoulder muscles in patients diagnosed with anterior glenohumeral instability. The patients who had instability demonstrated suppressed pectoralis major and biceps brachii mean reflexive activation, significantly slower biceps brachii reflex latency, and suppressed supraspinatus-subscapularis coactivation. The results suggest that in addition to the capsuloligamentous deficiency and proprioceptive deficits present in patients who have anterior glenohumeral instability, muscle activation alterations are also present. The suppressed rotator cuff coactivation, slower biceps brachii activation, and decreased pectoralis major and biceps brachii mean activation may contribute to the recurrent instability episodes seen in patients who have glenohumeral instability. To date, there is no research that specifically examines the effects of injury on shoulder muscle stiffness characteristics.

The altered neuromuscular control mechanisms seen in patients who have instability are believed to be related to altered joint function. For example, individuals who have multidirectional instability demonstrate proprioceptive deficits [49], neuromuscular alterations (altered muscle firing patterns) [56,58,59], and altered movement patterns [60,61]. The coexistence of these conditions in patients who have instability suggests strong association and potential cause-and-effect relationship among the conditions. The glenohumeral instability and the dysfunctional neuromuscular control may together contribute to the dysfunction associated with instability.

Sensorimotor Alterations with Rotator Cuff Disease

Sensorimotor alterations have been identified in patients who have various degrees of rotator cuff disease ranging from subacromial impingement to rotator cuff lesions. From a review of the literature, the most likely culprit of the sensorimotor dysfunction is the pain associated with the impingement or rotator cuff tear. Assessment of proprioception in patients who have rotator cuff disease has been limited. Machner and colleagues [62] demonstrated decreased kinesthesia in subjects diagnosed with unilateral stage II subacromial impingement. The authors theorized that the subacromial bursa was deficient in relaying the movement sense signals because of the compression and pain [62]. Safran and colleagues [63] demonstrated that throwers who have shoulder pain have proprioception deficits and suggested that increased nociceptor activity in the painful shoulder overrode proprioceptive input.

Muscle activation abnormalities associated with subacromial impingement and rotator cuff lesions have also been identified [64–69]. Common findings include altered activity of the primary humeral movers, decreased activity in the supraspinatus, infraspinatus, and subscapularis, decreased coactivation of the rotator cuff musculature, and suppressed scapular stabilization by the trapezius and serratus anterior muscles during elevation. Kelly and colleagues [66] assessed activation of the rotator cuff during functional tasks and demonstrated that patients who have painful rotator cuff tears exhibit activation alterations in muscles around the injured shoulder that may limit functional performance compared with both the asymptomatic side and shoulders of normal participants, suggesting that pain is the major contributor to the altered muscle activation patterns seen in patients who have rotator cuff tears. Bandholm and colleagues [68] induced experimental shoulder pain by a bolus injection of

6% hypertonic saline into the supraspinatus muscle of healthy participants and demonstrated altered activation of the middle deltoid and infraspinatus and lower trapezius. These results demonstrate the potent effect pain has on muscle activation patterns. Research using anesthesia models to examine the role of pain on shoulder function has demonstrated muscle activation patterns, strength, and movement patterns that better reflect normal muscle activation and movement in patients who have rotator cuff tears following lidocaine injection [70–73].

Like shoulder instability, the sensorimotor alterations associated with rotator cuff disease are believed to result in decreased function. For example, individuals who had subacromial impingement and rotator cuff tears demonstrated altered scapular movement patterns, including decreased scapular upward rotation, increased scapular anterior tipping, increased scapular retraction, and decreased scapulohumeral rhythm, during a functional overhead task [64,72,74,75]. Bandholm and colleagues [69] demonstrated deficits in force steadiness (defined as maintenance of submaximal isometric contraction) and maximum strength deficits in patients who had subacromial impingement or rotator cuff tears. Patients who have rotator cuff pathology have strength deficits in shoulder elevation and rotation movement patterns [71,76].

SUMMARY

The shoulder complex relies heavily on dynamic action of the musculature that is mediated by the sensorimotor system to maintain stability and allow for coordinated action by the four articulations involved with shoulder motion. When the shoulder sustains an injury, tissue pathology and pain result. Sensorimotor alterations also manifest, most likely a result of the tissue pathology and pain. Sensorimotor deficits in the form of proprioception and alteration in neuromuscular control have been demonstrated in shoulders with various degrees of instability and rotator cuff disease. The combination of the tissue pathology, pain, and sensorimotor alterations directly affect outcome following injury, and thus need to be addressed by the clinician treating the shoulder injury to fully restore function.

References

[1] Freedman L, Munro RR. Abduction of the arm in the scapular plane: scapular and glenohumeral movements. A roentgenographic study. J Bone Joint Surg Am 1966;48(8):1503–10.

[2] Harryman DT, Sidles JA, Harris SL, et al. The role of the rotator interval capsule in passive motion and stability of the shoulder. J Bone Joint Surg Am 1992;74(1):53–66.

[3] Levangie PK, Norkin CC. Joint structure and function: a comprehensive analysis. 3rd edition. Philadelphia: F.A. Davis Company; 2001.

[4] Saha A. Mechanism of shoulder movements and a plea for the recognition of "zero position" of the glenohumeral joint. Indian J Surg 1950;12:153–65.

[5] Doody SG, Freedman L, Waterland JC. Shoulder movements during abduction in the scapular plane. Arch Phys Med Rehabil 1970;51(10):595–604.

[6] Ludewig PM, Behrens SA, Meyer SM, et al. Three-dimensional clavicular motion during arm elevation: reliability and descriptive data. J Orthop Sports Phys Ther 2004;34(3):140–9.

[7] Sahara W, Sugamoto K, Murai M, et al. Three-dimensional clavicular and acromioclavicular rotations during arm abduction using vertically open MRI. J Orthop Res 2007;25(9): 1243–9.

[8] Harryman DT III, Sidles JA, Harris SL, et al. Laxity of the normal glenohumeral joint: a quantitative in-vivo assessment. J Shoulder Elbow Surg 1990;1:66–76.

[9] Lephart SM, Riemann BL, Fu F. Introduction to the sensorimotor system. In: Lephart SM, Fu FH, editors. Proprioception and neuromuscular control in joint stability. Champaign (IL): Human Kinetics; 2000. p. xvii–xiv.

[10] Grigg P. Peripheral neural mechanism in proprioception. J Sport Rehabil 1994;3:2–17.

[11] Kikuchi T. Histological studies on the sensory innervation of the shoulder joint. Journal of Iwate Medical Association 1968;20:554–67.

[12] Vangsness CT, Ennis M, Taylor JG, et al. Neural anatomy of the glenohumeral ligaments, labrum, and subacromial bursa. Arthroscopy 1995;11(2):180–4.

[13] Nyland JA, Caborn DN, Johnson DL. The human glenohumeral joint: a proprioceptive and stability alliance. Knee Surg Sports Traumatol Arthrosc 1998;6(1):50–61.

[14] Riemann BL, Lephart SM. The sensorimotor system, part 1: the physiological basis of functional joint stability. J Athl Train 2002;37(1):71–9.

[15] Riemann BL, Lephart SM. The sensorimotor system, part 2: the role of proprioception in motor control and functional joint stability. J Athl Train 2002;37(1):80–4.

[16] Myers JB, Lephart SM. The role of the sensorimotor system in the athletic shoulder. J Athl Train 2000;35(3):351–63.

[17] Myers JB, Lephart SM. Sensorimotor deficits contributing to glenohumeral instability. Clin Orthop Relat Res 2002;400:98–104.

[18] Lephart SM, Kocher MS. The role of exercise in the prevention of shoulder disorders. In: Matsen FA, Fu FH, Hawkins RJ, editors. The shoulder: a balance of mobility and stability. Presented at AAOS. San Francisco, February 19, 2003.

[19] Inman VT, Saunders JR, Abbott JC. Observations on the function of the shoulder joint. J Bone Joint Surg 1944;26:1–30.

[20] Lephart SM, Henry TJ. The physiological basis for open and closed kinetic chain rehabilitation for the upper extremity. J Sport Rehabil 1996;5:71–87.

[21] Cleland J. On the actions of muscles passing over more than one joint. J Anat Physiol 1866;1:85–93.

[22] Wilk KE, Arrigo CA. Current concepts in the rehabilitation of the athletic shoulder. J Orthop Sports Phys Ther 1993;18(1):365–78.

[23] Peat M, Culham E. Functional anatomy of the shoulder complex. In: Andrews JR, Wilk KE, editors. The athlete's shoulder. 1st edition. New York: Churchill Livingstone; 1994. p. 1–13.

[24] Jerosch J, Steinbeck J, Schrode M, et al. Intraoperative EMG-ableitungbein reizug de glenohumeralin glenehkapsel. Unfallchirurg 1995;98:580–5.

[25] Schutte MJ, Dabezies EJ, Zimny ML, et al. Neural anatomy of the human anterior cruciate ligament. J Bone Joint Surg 1987;69A:243–7.

[26] Johansson H, Sjolander P, Sojka P. A sensory role for the cruciate ligaments. Clin Orthop 1991;268:161–78.

[27] Johansson H. Role of knee ligaments in proprioception and regulation of muscle stiffness. J Electromyogr Kinesiol 1991;3:158–79.

[28] Johansson H, Pedersen J, Bergenheim M, et al. Peripheral afferents of the knee: their effects on central mechanisms regulating muscle stiffness, joint stability, and proprioception and coordination. In: Lephart SM, Fu FH, editors. Proprioception and neuromuscular control in joint stability. Champaign (IL): Human Kinetics; 2000. p. 5–22.

[29] Oatis CA. The use of a mechanical model to describe the stiffness and dampening characteristics of the knee joint in healthy adults. Phys Ther 1993;73(11):740–9.

[30] Akazawa K, Aldridge JW, Steeves JD, et al. Modulation of stretch reflexes during locomotion in the mesencephalic cat. J Physiol (London) 1982;329:553–67.

[31] Akazawa K, Milner TE, Stein RB. Modulation of reflex EMG and stiffness in response to stretch of human finger muscles. J Neurophysiol 1983;49:16–27.

[32] Blanpied P, Smidt GL. Human plantarflexor stiffness to multiple single stretch trials. J Biomech 1992;25(1):29–39.

[33] McNair PJ, Wood GA, Marshall RN. Stiffness of the hamstring muscles and its relationship to function in anterior cruciate deficient individuals. Clin Biomech 1992;7:131–7.

[34] Sinkjaer T, Toft E, Andreassen S, et al. Muscle stiffness in human ankle dorsiflexors: Intrinsic and reflex components. J Neurophysiol 1988;60(3):1110–21.

[35] Sinkjaer T, Hayashi R. Regulation of wrist stiffness by the stretch reflex. J Biomech 1989;22:1133–40.

[36] Loeb GE, Brown IE, Cheng EJ. A hierarchical foundation for models of sensorimotor control. Exp Brain Res 1999;126(1):1–18.

[37] Wilson GJ, Wood GA, Elliott BC. The relationship between stiffness of the musculature and static flexibility: an alternative explanation for the occurrence of muscular injury. Int J Sports Med 1991;12(4):403–7.

[38] Wilkie DR. The relation between force and velocity in human muscle. J Physiol (London) 1949;110:249–80.

[39] Morgan DL. Separation of active and passive components of short range stiffness of muscle. Am J Physiol 1977;232(1):45–9.

[40] Ma SP, Zahalak GI. The mechanical response of the active human triceps brachii to very rapid stretch and shortening. J Biomech 1985;18(8):585–98.

[41] Zhang L, Portland GH, Wang G, et al. Stiffness, viscosity, and upper limb inertia about the glenohumeral abduction axis. J Orthop Res 2000;18:94–100.

[42] Weiss PL, Hunter LW, Kearney RE. Human ankle joint stiffness over the full range of muscle activation levels. J Biomech 1988;21:539–44.

[43] Johansson H, Sjolander P, Sojka P, et al. Reflex actions on the gamma muscle spindle systems of muscle activity at the knee joint elicited by stretch of the posterior cruciate ligament. Neurological Orthopedics 1989;8:9–21.

[44] Johansson H, Sjolander P, Sojka P. Receptors in the knee joint ligaments and their role in the biomechanics of the joint. CRC Crit Rev Biomed Eng 1991;18:341–68.

[45] Tibone JE, Fechter J, Kao JT. Evaluation of a proprioception pathway in patients with stable and unstable shoulders with cortical evoked potentials. J Shoulder Elbow Surg 1997;6(5):440–3.

[46] Forwell LA, Carnahan H. Proprioception during manual aiming in individuals with shoulder instability and controls. J Orthop Sports Phys Ther 1996;23(2):111–9.

[47] Lephart SM, Warner JP, Borsa PA, et al. Proprioception of the shoulder joint in healthy, unstable, and surgically repaired shoulders. J Shoulder Elbow Surg 1994;3(6):371–80.

[48] Zuckerman JD, Gallagher MA, Cuomo F, et al. The effect of instability and subsequent anterior shoulder repair on proprioceptive ability. J Shoulder Elbow Surg 2003;12(2):105–9.

[49] Barden JM, Balyk R, Raso VJ, et al. Dynamic upper limb proprioception in multidirectional shoulder instability. Clin Orthop 2004;420:181–9.

[50] Aydin T, Yildiz Y, Yanmis I, et al. Shoulder proprioception: a comparison between the shoulder joint in healthy and surgically repaired shoulders. Arch Orthop Trauma Surg 2001;121(7):422–5.

[51] Lephart SM, Myers JB, Bradley JP, et al. Shoulder proprioception and function following thermal capsulorrhaphy. Arthroscopy 2002;18(7):770–8.

[52] Potzl W, Thorwesten L, Gotze C, et al. Proprioception of the shoulder joint after surgical repair for instability: a long-term follow-up study. Am J Sports Med 2004;32(2):425–30.

[53] Fremerey R, Bosch U, Freitag N, et al. Proprioception and EMG pattern after capsulolabral reconstruction in shoulder instability: a clinical and experimental study. Knee Surg Sports Traumatol Arthrosc 2006;14(12):1315–20.

[54] Myers JB, Ju YY, Hwang JH, et al. Reflexive muscle activation alterations in shoulders with anterior glenohumeral instability. Am J Sports Med 2004;32(4):1013–21.

[55] McMahon PJ, Jobe FW, Pink MM, et al. Comparative electromyographic analysis of shoulder muscles during planar motions: anterior glenohumeral instability versus normal. J Shoulder Elbow Surg 1996;5(2 Pt 1):118–23.

[56] Kronberg M, Brostrom LA, Nemeth G. Differences in shoulder muscle activity between patients with generalized joint laxity and normal controls. Clin Orthop 1991;269:181–92.

[57] Glousman R, Jobe F, Tibone J, et al. Dynamic electromyographic analysis of the throwing shoulder with glenohumeral instability. J Bone Joint Surg Am 1988;70(2):220–6.

[58] Barden JM, Balyk R, Raso VJ, et al. Atypical shoulder muscle activation in multidirectional instability. Clin Neurophysiol 2005;116(8):1846–57.

[59] Morris AD, Kemp GJ, Frostick SP. Shoulder electromyography in multidirectional instability. J Shoulder Elbow Surg 2004;13(1):24–9.

[60] Matias R, Pascoal AG. The unstable shoulder in arm elevation: a three-dimensional and electromyographic study in subjects with glenohumeral instability. Clin Biomech 2006; 21(Suppl 1):S52–8.

[61] Ogston JB, Ludewig PM. Differences in 3-dimensional shoulder kinematics between persons with multidirectional instability and asymptomatic controls. Am J Sports Med 2007;35(8): 1361–70.

[62] Machner A, Merk H, Becker R, et al. Kinesthetic sense of the shoulder in patients with impingement syndrome. Acta Orthop Scand 2003;74(1):85–8.

[63] Safran MR, Borsa PA, Lephart SM, et al. Shoulder proprioception in baseball pitchers. J Shoulder Elbow Surg 2001;10(5):438–44.

[64] Ludewig PM, Cook TM. Alterations in shoulder kinematics and associated muscle activity in people with symptoms of shoulder impingement. Phys Ther 2000;80(3):276–91.

[65] Reddy AS, Mohr KJ, Pink MM, et al. Electromyographic analysis of the deltoid and rotator cuff muscles in persons with subacromial impingement. J Shoulder Elbow Surg 2000;9(6):519–23.

[66] Kelly BT, Williams RJ, Cordasco FA, et al. Differential patterns of muscle activation in patients with symptomatic and asymptomatic rotator cuff tears. J Shoulder Elbow Surg 2005;14(2): 165–71.

[67] Myers JB, Hwang JH, Pasquale MR, et al. Shoulder muscle coactivation alterations in patients with subacromial impingement. Paper presented at the: 2003 American College of Sports Medicine annual meeting. San Francisco, May 28–June 1, 2003.

[68] Bandholm T, Rasmussen L, Aagaard P, et al. Effects of experimental muscle pain on shoulder-abduction force steadiness and muscle activity in healthy subjects. Eur J Appl Physiol 2008;102:643–50.

[69] Bandholm T, Rasmussen L, Aagaard P, et al. Force steadiness, muscle activity, and maximal muscle strength in subjects with subacromial impingement syndrome. Muscle Nerve 2006;34(5):631–9.

[70] Kirschenbaum D, Coyle MP Jr, Leddy JP, et al. Shoulder strength with rotator cuff tears. Pre- and postoperative analysis. Clin Orthop 1993;(288):174–8.

[71] Ben-Yishay A, Zuckerman JD, Gallagher M, et al. Pain inhibition of shoulder strength in patients with impingement syndrome. Orthopedics 1994;17(8):685–8.

[72] Scibek JS, Mell AG, Downie BK, et al. Shoulder kinematics in patients with full-thickness rotator cuff tears after a subacromial injection. J Shoulder Elbow Surg 2007;17:172–81.

[73] Steenbrink F, de Groot JH, Veeger HE, et al. Pathological muscle activation patterns in patients with massive rotator cuff tears, with and without subacromial anesthetics. Man Ther 2006;11(3):231–7.

[74] Lukasiewicz AC, McClure P, Michener L, et al. Comparison of 3-dimensional scapular position and orientation between subjects with and without shoulder impingement. J Orthop Sports Phys Ther 1999;29(10):574–83 [discussion: 584–576].

[75] Ludewig PM, Cook TM. Translations of the humerus in persons with shoulder impingement symptoms. J Orthop Sports Phys Ther 2002;32(6):248–59.

[76] Rokito AS, Zuckerman JD, Gallagher MA, et al. Strength after surgical repair of the rotator cuff. J Shoulder Elbow Surg 1996;5(1):12–7.

Clin Sports Med 27 (2008) 491–505

CLINICS IN SPORTS MEDICINE

ELSEVIER
SAUNDERS

Evaluation of Health-Related Quality of Life in Patients with Shoulder Pain: Are We Doing the Best We Can?

Lori A. Michener, PhD, PT, ATC, SCS[a],*,
Alison R. Snyder, PhD, ATC[b]

[a]Department of Physical Therapy, Virginia Commonwealth University, Medical College
of Virginia Campus, P.O. Box 980224, Rm 100, 12th and Broad Streets, Richmond, VA 23298, USA
[b]Department of Interdisciplinary Health Sciences, Athletic Training Program, A.T. Still University,
5850 E. Still Circle, Mesa, AZ 85206, USA

The evaluation of health-related quality of life (HRQOL) in people suffering from shoulder pain is critical for the comprehensive assessment of the impact of the disease on the person's health status. HRQOL refers to "the physical, psychologic, and social domains of health, seen as distinct areas that are influenced by a person's experiences, beliefs, expectation, and perceptions" [1]. Measurement of HRQOL using appropriate patient-oriented outcome instruments is helpful in guiding treatment decision-making, determining prognosis, and making judgments as to the response to treatment. Traditionally, clinicians have emphasized the use of clinician-based measures of outcome, such as range-of-motion and strength, as opposed to patient-based outcomes. One reason for the focus on clinician-based outcome measures is due to their long-standing use and familiarity [2]. Recently patient-centered whole-person health care has been recognized and promoted by a variety of health care professionals and organizations [3–6]. This recognition has translated into increased development and use of patient-oriented outcome instruments to assess shoulder function and disability in individuals with high physical demand on their shoulders [7–10]. Patient-centered care requires the identification and respect of individual patient differences, preferences, values, and needs [4]. Similarly, a whole-person approach to care necessitates the evaluation of all components of the health spectrum, from pathophysiology to disability, best obtained through patient-based measures of outcome [6,11,12].

Unlike clinician-based measures that emphasize pathophysiology and impairments, patient-based outcome measures assess the functional status and level of disability of the patient from the patient's perspective and provide information regarding what is important to him or her. Examples of patient-based outcomes

*Corresponding author. E-mail address: lamichen@vcu.edu (L.A. Michener).

0278-5919/08/$ – see front matter
doi:10.1016/j.csm.2008.03.001

include measures of return-to-play; of functional ability to perform daily activities, such as dressing; of ability to perform work and sport activities; and of patient satisfaction [13]. Without patient-based measures, it is impossible to evaluate the whole person and, thus, difficult to ascertain the true impact of an injury, disease, or condition on a person's overall health status. Lack of patient-based measures leaves the clinician to focus on impairments and to assume that impairments are directly related to functional limitations and disability, which may not be the case [13–15]. For example, a person may have an obvious impairment, such as reduced shoulder flexion range-of-motion. However, if this reduction in shoulder motion does not negatively impact the ability to perform activities of daily living, work tasks, or sport activities, then it is not classified as a disability. Clinician-based measures are more likely to be poor indicators of functional ability and psychologic health status [2].

The shift from solely clinician-based to a combination of clinician- plus patient-based assessment is critical to broadly and accurately assess the impact of a disease on the patient's HRQOL. Unfortunately, patient-based information has been less valued and performed to a lesser extent in clinical practice because of the assumption that it is difficult to measure patient views accurately and reliably [2,10]. If patient-based measures demonstrate adequate reliability and validity for their intended clinical purpose, then they are suitable for use. It has become increasingly clear that patient input is necessary to adequately assess the effect of disease, such as a shoulder disorder, to determine prognosis, and for the evaluation of outcomes of treatment interventions and programs [2,16–18]. Evidence indicates that patient-oriented measures are important because the patient perspective is the best estimate of HRQOL [2,17,19]. Furthermore, there are likely discrepancies between the patient perception of an injury and the severity of the condition as evaluated through clinician-based outcome measures [20].

This article provides an understanding of patient-based shoulder outcome tools and the conceptual framework of disablement models from which the patient-based outcome tools are based. To allow for the evaluation of function, disability, and HRQOL in patients suffering from shoulder pain and in particular in those whose shoulders have high physical demands, shoulder self-report patient-oriented outcome tools must become standard of practice.

DISABLEMENT MODELS

Disablement models provide a conceptual framework for a whole-person approach to health care. Generically, disablement models are organized at the origin, organ, person, and societal levels [21]. As a conceptual framework, disablement models define concepts and relationships related to disability and assist with generating hypotheses amongst the framework variables [22]. Disablement models assist with the care of patients with shoulder dysfunctions and pain by providing a conceptual framework that indicates the components necessary to examine, measure, and comprehensively assess the impact of disease. Since the mid 1960s, several disablement models have been created or modified, with most attention given to the Nagi Model of Disablement [23] and the International Classification of Functioning, Disability, and Health (ICF) [24,25].

Nagi Model of Disablement

Nagi, a sociologist, developed the first disablement model based on his understanding that disability was influenced by more than the individual person and that such factors as family, community, and society have the potential to impact disability as well [21,23]. According to the Nagi model, disablement is defined by active pathology, impairments, functional limitations, and disability (Fig. 1) [23]. In brief, active pathology refers to the process of an injury, condition, or disease and often is described by diagnoses, whereas impairments relate to the anatomic or physiologic abnormalities resulting from the particular injury, condition, or disease and are often quantified by clinician-based measures (eg, range-of-motion, strength, and gait assessment) [23]. While functional limitations and disability both relate to body functioning, disability implies a social context to the activity whereas functional limitations implies no such context. The result of the Nagi model is that the consequence of disease (active pathology) is explained in terms of its effect on body functions (impairments), the person's ability to complete functional tasks (functional limitations), and the person's ability to fulfill his or her life roles (disability) [26].

Although the Nagi model is influential in highlighting the complexity in disablement and in focusing attention on the individual and his or her environment, more recent models, including the ICF, have attempted to expand upon the Nagi model by more completely encompassing the dimensions of disability and the additional factors that impact disablement.

World Health Organization's International Classification of Functioning, Disability, and Health

In 2001, the World Health Organization released its most recent disablement model, the ICF [24,25,27], which is a revision of the International Classification of Impairments, Disability, and Handicap (ICIDH) (Fig. 2). Since its release, health care organizations, such as the Institute of Medicine [28], and professional organizations, such as those representing speech pathologists [29], physical therapists [30,31], and athletic trainers [6], have considered the role of the ICF in their institutions and professions. Discussion of the ICF is warranted

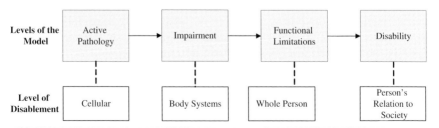

Fig. 1. Nagi model.

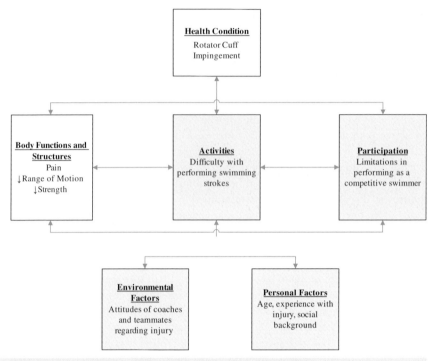

Fig. 2. ICF model. Shaded areas indicate components of HRQOL.

because its eventual success in enhancing patient care requires an understanding of its theories and components. The ICF was created through a collaboration of individuals from around the world with the goal of creating a comprehensive model of disablement that would provide a standard language for disability, create a scientific basis for understanding and studying health and health-related outcomes, and allow comparisons of data among countries and health care disciplines [25].

One of the main differences between the ICF and the Nagi model is the terminology used to describe disablement. However, the definitions of the components remain relatively similar. For example, active pathology in the Nagi model most closely relates to health condition in the ICF, which refers to the actual diagnosis of the injury, condition, or disease. Body functions and structures refer to the physiologic functioning of body systems and the anatomic parts of the body and are often described in terms of impairments. Activities, as defined by the ICF, are those done at an individual level, whereas participation implies involvement in life situations, and these terms are most similar to Nagi's functional limitations and disability, respectively. In the ICF, however, functioning and disability are overarching terms rather than categories. Functioning explains all body functions, activities, and participation, whereas disability refers to impairments, activity limitations, and participation restrictions

[25]. The addition of health-related domains creates a more comprehensive framework for assessing health status because it identifies the environment and personal factors as having the potential to influence all of the other constructs in the model [25]. For example, a competitive swimmer who suffers from rotator cuff impingement (health condition) may present with pain, reduced range-of-motion, and decreased strength in the shoulder region (body functions and structures) (see Fig. 2). Limitations in activity and participation are categorized by the athlete's decreased ability to perform swimming strokes, which may result in the inability to compete in scheduled swim meets. Additionally, environmental factors, such as a coach's attitude about the injured athlete, and personal factors, such as age, experience as a patient, and social background, may also influence the disablement level of the athlete. It is important to note that HRQOL is evaluated when the combination of information from activities and participation, environmental factors, and personal factors are considered, which necessitates the gathering of information from a variety of disablement model constructs (shaded areas of Fig. 2).

One of the benefits of using a disablement model, such as the ICF, is that the framework helps to increase understanding about a patient's condition from a whole-person point of view [32]. Additionally, implementing patient-based outcome measures to evaluate the specific components of disablement creates a patient-centered approach to care. The challenge, then, is in selecting meaningful and appropriate measures of outcome that evaluate activities, participation, and, ultimately, HRQOL in those with high physical demands on the shoulder suffering from shoulder dysfunction and pain.

PATIENT-ORIENTED OUTCOME TOOLS FOR SHOULDER PAIN

The measurement of activities, participation, and HRQOL can be accomplished by direct observation or by patient report. Direct observation will likely not allow for a comprehensive assessment because of the large amount of time and diversity of measurements needed to evaluate all meaningful activities required daily for a given individual. Patient-oriented outcome tools provide a quick and efficient method of measuring activities and participation and of overall HRQOL. Before choosing a scale or outcome tool, many factors need to be considered (Table 1).

Multi-Item Format Versus Single-Item Format

Questionnaires or instruments used to evaluate disablement constructs, including activities, participation, or overall HRQOL, come in a variety of formats. In general, instruments are broadly classified as either multi-item or single-item scales. Multi-item scales are either designed to measure one unified construct, such as activities, or are designed to measure a combination of multiple constructs, such as body structure and functions (eg, the measurement of pain), activities, participation, and/or overall HRQOL. This distinction is crucial because all patient-oriented outcome measures do not evaluate the same constructs or even dimensions of constructs. For example, the Disabilities of the

Table 1
Description of commonly used patient self-report outcomes for the shoulder

Scale	Type	Number of questions (ICF dimensions)	Score	Answer format	Number of questions related to high-demand shoulder activities
Short-Form 36 (SF-36)	Generic; multi-item	36	2 component scores; 8 construct scores	5-option Likert	None
Disabilities of the Arm, Shoulder, Hand (DASH)	Upper limb; multi-item	30 (5 body functions and structures; 25 activities and participation)	0–100 (0 = no disability)	5-option Likert	7 (2 specific to sports)
American Shoulder and Elbow Surgeons Patient Assessment (ASES) Self-Report Section	Shoulder; multi-item	11 (1 body functions and structures ; 10 activities and participation)	0–100 (100 = no disability)	Pain: 10-cm visual analog scale; activities and participation: 4-option Likert	5 (2 specific to sports)
Simple Shoulder Test (SST)	Shoulder; multi-item	12 (1 body functions and structures ; 11 activities and participation)	0–12 (12 = no disability)	Dichotomous yes/no	6 (2 specific to sports)
Shoulder Disability Questionnaire, Netherlands Version (SDQ)	Shoulder	16 (16 activities and participation)	0–100 (100 = no disability)	Dichotomous yes/no	1 (none specific to sports)
Constant Self-Report Section	Shoulder	5 (1 body functions and structures ; 4 activities and participation)	0–35 (35 = no disability)	Pain: 4-option Likert; activities and participation: 2- or 5-option Likert	2 (1 specific to sports)
Constant Clinician Section	Shoulder	None (measurements taken for range-of-motion and strength)	0–65 (65 = full range and strength)	Range-of-motion: 4-option Likert; strength: abduction-resisted pounds up to 25 lb	Not applicable
Pain: numeric pain rating scale	Single item	1 (1 body functions and structures)	0–10 (0 = no pain)	11-point numeric rating	None
Patient satisfaction: shoulder use	Single item	1 (1 activities and participation)	0–10 (0 = not satisfied)	11-point numeric rating	None

Arm, Shoulder and Hand (DASH) [33] measures items from three parts of the ICF model: (1) symptoms of pain, tingling, and numbness; (2) difficulty in completing daily tasks, such as putting on a pullover sweater; and (3) the impact the shoulder disorder has on social activities. The clinician and researcher must have a firm understanding of the underlying dimensions that a multi-item scale is measuring to allow for proper interpretation and application of the scores.

Single-item questions, also typically referred to as global questions, contain just one question, which is designed to globally assess a single construct. A numeric pain rating scale is a single-item question that asks the patient to rate his or her pain on a scale of 0 to 10, using the anchors of "no pain" and "worse pain imaginable." An example of a single question aimed at assessing shoulder disability is the Single Assessment Numeric Evaluation (SANE), which asks: "How would you rate your shoulder today as a percentage of normal (0–100% scale with 100% being normal)?" [34].

Multi-item and single-item scales can be used together to measure disability in patients with shoulder pain, as both have distinct advantages and disadvantages. Multi-item scales for the shoulder, such as the DASH, take longer to complete and score as compared with the single question, which likely takes less than 1 minute. However, multi-item scales make up for their length with their ability to assess the multidimensional impact of a shoulder disorder by containing a variety of items for the assessment of daily activities and participation, and often capture what individuals want or need to do on a daily basis. Single questions, such as the SANE, are good for obtaining a general assessment of the construct of shoulder disability but are limited in their ability to comprehensively evaluate the complex phenomenon of shoulder disability. When patients are asked a single question, such as the SANE, they may focus on just one activity, instead of considering all the activities they are required to do with their shoulder. This can result in a single item score that does not accurately reflect the overall level of shoulder disability. Moreover, the single-item scale may be unable to detect change over time when true change in disability has occurred..

Answer Format Options

There are multiple answer formats for patient self-report questionnaires. The most commonly used answer formats are a visual analog scale, the Likert scale with a number of response options, the dichotomous response option, and a numeric rating scale. The visual analog scale is a line, typically 100 mm long, with qualifying anchor statements for each end of the scale. The patient places a mark on scale, and then the distance from one of the ends is measured. A Likert scale answer format typically has three or five response options, while dichotomous response options have two options of typically "yes" or "no." Lastly, a numeric rating scale is most commonly an 11-point scale, asking the patient to rate an activity, their level of pain, or something else. Each answer format has its own advantages and disadvantages in terms of time imposed on the patient and the clinician/researcher in scoring responses and in terms of the reliability, sensitivity, or responsiveness of the scale to detect meaningful change.

Practicality

A scale must be practical for use in a clinical setting. If it is not, clinicians and researchers will not universally adopt it. When a scale is used clinically in the management of patients, the results of the scale should be reviewed with the patient. A questionnaire should be easy to read and understand, short enough to be feasible but long enough to be comprehensive in measuring the construct, and easy to score and interpret. Generally, shorter scales are less of a burden for patients, take less time to score, and are more economical because they require less time and paper for completion [35]. These practical factors, however, cannot outweigh the purpose and needs of the clinician or researcher.

Purpose of the Scale

The intended use of the scale must be considered when selecting an instrument. Disability scales are used to determine prognosis, discriminate at a single point in time, and assess change over time in disability [36]. Before using a scale, evidence should demonstrate that the scale can serve its intended purpose. For example, a scale that is designed to measure change in disability over time should demonstrate its ability to be responsive and sensitive to change. A thorough investigation of the measurement properties is necessary before acceptance and use of a scale.

Psychometric Properties of Scales

Psychometric or measurement properties of any tool must be established before use. At a minimum, a scale should be tested in a sample group of patients similar to those for whom the scale is intended to determine its test-retest reliability, internal consistency, content and construct validity, error estimates, and responsiveness [37]. Reliability is the accuracy or precision of a scale, with test-retest reliability as the ability of the scale to generate the same score over time in individuals whose shoulder disability has not changed. A value of 0.75 for an intraclass correlation coefficient or kappa coefficient is considered an acceptable level of reliability [38]. Internal consistency is the homogeneity or similarity of the items that form the scale, which is reported with a Cronbach's alpha coefficient. Scores range from 0 to 1, with coefficients closer to 1 indicating a substantial relationship or correlation among the items on the scale [37,39].

Error estimates are arguably the most useful measurement properties. Error estimates are used to make judgments regarding the scale's results of a single score or a change in score over time. The standard error of the measure (SEM) is an estimate of the error of a score when a patient completes a score just one time. The minimal detectable change (MDC) is the error associated with two scores, or change scores. The SEM and MDC are calculated thus:

SEM = [standard deviation (from the study on internal consistency) × square root of (1−Cronbach's alpha)]

MDC = [standard deviation (from the study on test-retest reliability) × square root of $(1-ICC)$] × square root of 2.

The SEM and MDC are calculated with 68% confidence bounds. To calculate the 90% or 95% confidence bounds, multiply the SEM or MDC by the appropriate z-score (90% confidence bound: 1.64; 95% confidence bound: 1.96). These values can then be used to interpret scores for individual patients [10].

Validity assessment is important to determine if the scale is measuring what it purports to measure and the extent by which a meaningful interpretation can be made about the scores. Content validity and construct validity are the minimal aspects that should be reported about the scale. Responsiveness, as an aspect of validity, is the ability of a scale to measure clinical change [36]. These statistics indicate the ability to detect clinical change in groups of patients and are commonly reported as standardized response means and effect sizes.

Measurement of High-Demand Activities and Participation Related to the Shoulder

A plethora of shoulder scales have been developed and examined with respect to measurement properties. However, no shoulder scale has been developed and tested that is condition-specific to the shoulder and specific to high-demand activities and participation or designed specifically for those participating in sports [8]. Most shoulder scales do contain one or more items specific to the performance of high-demand activities, such as "reaching overhead," "carrying heavy objects" and "lift a gallon container to shoulder level." All shoulder scales contain a single item to measure the ability to participate in sports or work activities. The DASH contains an optional module to measure ability to participate in sports or performing arts. Previous studies that have reviewed or examined the ability of shoulder scales to measure athlete function and disability describe a likely lack of specificity of the scales to measure shoulder disability in athletes [8,9,40,41]. Presently no studies report measurement properties or the ability of a condition-specific shoulder scale to measure shoulder disability in athletes or in patients with shoulder pain and high-level shoulder demand.

Scales

Numerous self-report scales measure function and disability of the shoulder and general HRQOL. This article does not attempt to present all of these scales. Rather, the article presents a couple of scales and describes their ability to measure shoulder activities and participation. Additionally, the ability of the scales to measure high-demand work and recreation is discussed. Generic measures are designed to measure HRQOL for any health condition, while specific scales are designed to assess a specific condition or region of the body, such as the shoulder (condition) or arm (region). There are also disease-specific scales designed to assess a specific disease, such as shoulder instability.

The medical outcomes trust short-form 36

The Medical Outcomes Trust Short-Form 36 (SF-36) is a generic measure designed to assess HRQOL [42,43]. The SF-36 is a commonly used generic health-status measure with 10 constructs, 8 subscales and 2 summary scores. The subscales are (1) physical function; (2) role limitations due to physical health; (3) role limitations due to emotional problems; (4) vitality, energy, and fatigue; (5) mental health; (6) social functioning; (7) bodily pain; and (8) general health. Higher scores on the subscales are indicative of less disability, while the 2 summary scores have established normative values of a mean of 50 points [42,43]. The SF-36 has been shown to be a reliable, valid, and responsive generic measure of the health of patients with musculoskeletal conditions [44].

The disabilities of the arm, shoulder and hand questionnaire
The DASH is a 30-question region-specific self-report outcome tool for upper extremity disability [33]. The DASH considers both extremities as a single unit by asking the patient to answer based on ability to perform the tasks "regardless of how you perform the task," stating that "it doesn't matter which hand or arm you use to perform the activity." The DASH has been extensively tested for adequacy of measurement properties [33,45–49].

The American shoulder and elbow surgeons patient self-report section
The American Shoulder and Elbow Surgeons Patient Self-Report Section (ASES), developed by the American Shoulder and Elbow Surgeons [50], is an 11-question scale that is condition-specific to the shoulder. It contains two sections, one for pain and one for activities and participation. One unique aspect of the ASES is that it asks the patient to consider the right or left shoulder when considering the level of difficulty with daily tasks. The ASES has demonstrated reliability, validity, and the ability to detect meaningful change [51–55].

The simple shoulder test
The Simple Shoulder Test (SST) was developed by a group of orthopedic surgeons with specialization in the shoulder [56]. It contains 12 items with dichotomous response options. Because the SST has this dichotomous response option, it may not be able to detect small but clinically important changes in patient disability status or to discriminate among levels of disability [9]. Evidence indicates that the SST has adequate measurement properties and is responsive [51,57–59].

The shoulder disability questionnaire
The Shoulder Disability Questionnaire, Netherlands Version (SDQ), was developed to assess changes in pain-related disability of the shoulder [60]. It contains 16 items with dichotomous response options of "yes" and "no" and has been extensively studied in patients with shoulder pain and disability [60–63]. It was developed to measure change over time of pain-related disability of the shoulder, and has been demonstrated to be reliable, responsive, and have discriminate validity. One criticism of the SDQ is that it focuses on pain-related disability and does not address difficulty with activities and participation.

The constant score

The Constant score [64] is likely one of the most widely used shoulder instruments for the functional assessment of the shoulder. It contains two sections, one patient self-report and one clinician report. The patient report section contains just five questions. These are related to pain, work, sport, sleep, and positioning of the arm. These items are weighted, with pain representing 15% of the overall score and the other four function questions combined representing 20% of the total score. However, it has not been demonstrated that the four function questions adequately sample and represent the construct of shoulder disability. The clinician-based measures are range-of-motion, representing 40% of the score, and strength, representing 25% of the total score. The Constant score is a combined measure of body structure and function, activities, and participation, and the score is weighted in favor of the body structure and function components.

Patient satisfaction

Patient satisfaction has two underlying frameworks: (1) patient satisfaction with delivery of care and (2) patient satisfaction with the use of the injured body part. Patient satisfaction with use of the injured shoulder has been measured using an 11-point rating scale. A single question regarding the patient's satisfaction with shoulder function is anchored with "not satisfied" and "very satisfied." The test-retest reliability of this satisfaction rating has been established as excellent (intraclass correlation coefficient 0.93) in patients with shoulder pain [65].

Pain

Pain is considered a measure of impairment of body structure and function. However, if an outcome tool contains a question that asks about pain during an activity (eg, "Do you have pain when pulling on a sweater overhead?"), that question is classified as an Activity or Participation item. A numeric pain rating scale in various forms and as a part of other shoulder scales has been demonstrated to be reliable [54,65].

SUMMARY

Currently self-report outcome tools are used inconsistently in the clinic to assess patients [66]. This is unfortunate because the impact of a shoulder disorder cannot be fully understood without the assessment of shoulder disability. It is imperative that activities and participation be measured to ensure comprehensive assessment across the ICF disablement model. A wide variety of outcome tools are available that demonstrate acceptable levels of measurement properties and are appropriate for use for virtually every patient with a shoulder disorder. It is unclear why these tools are not being used routinely. In assessing patients with high-level shoulder demands, scales should contain items to measure high-demand activities or sport activities. It may be best to use a couple of scales, such as the DASH, DASH sport module, patient satisfaction, and pain scales to adequately assess the impact of a shoulder disorder. Currently, there is no general agreement as to the core set of outcome measures to use for patients with shoulder disorders. Future work is needed to develop a consensus on the core set of outcome measures for comprehensively assessing shoulder disorders.

References

[1] Testa MA, Simonson DC. Assessment of quality-of-life outcomes. N Engl J Med 1996;334(13):835–40.

[2] Kirkley A, Griffin S. Development of disease-specific quality of life measurement tools. Arthroscopy 2003;19(10):1121–8.

[3] Eechaute C, Vaes P, Van Aerschot L, et al. The clinimetric qualities of patient-assessed instruments for measuring chronic ankle instability: a systematic review. BMC Musculoskelet Disord 2007;8:6.

[4] Institute of Medicine. Health professions education: a bridge to quality. Washington, DC: Institute of Medicine; 2003.

[5] Pew Health Professions Commission. Critical challenges: revitalizing the health professions for the twenty-first century. Pew Charitable Trust; 1995.

[6] Snyder AR, Parsons JT, Valovich McLeod TC, et al. Utilizing disablement models and clinical outcomes assessment to enable evidence-based athletic training pracitce: part I—disablement models. J Athl Train, in Press.

[7] Bot SD, Terwee CB, van der Windt DA, et al. Clinimetric evaluation of shoulder disability questionnaires: a systematic review of the literature. Ann Rheum Dis 2004;63(4):335–41.

[8] Fayad F, Mace Y, Lefevre-Colau MM, et al. [Measurement of shoulder disability in the athlete: a systematic review.] Ann Readapt Med Phys 2004;47(6):389–95 [in French].

[9] Kirkley A, Griffin S, Dainty K. Scoring systems for the functional assessment of the shoulder. Arthroscopy 2003;19(10):1109–20.

[10] Michener LA, Leggin BG. A review of self-report scales for the assessment of functional limitation and disability of the shoulder. J Hand Ther 2001;14(2):68–76.

[11] Snyder AR, Valovich McLeod TC, Sauers EL. Defining, valuing, and teaching clinical outcomes assessment in professional and post-professional athletic training education programs. Athletic Training Education Journal 2007;2(Apr–Jun):1–11.

[12] Valovich McLeod TC, Snyder AR, Parsons JT, et al. Utilizing disablement models and clinical outcomes assessment to enable evidence-based athletic training practice: part II—clinical outcomes assessment. J Ath Train, in press.

[13] Binkley J. Measurement of functional status, progress and outcome in orthopaedic clinical practice. Orthopaedic Physical Therapy Practice 1999;11:14–21.

[14] Cross KM, Worrell TW, Leslie JE, et al. The relationship between self-reported and clinical measures and the number of days to return to sport following acute lateral ankle sprains. J Orthop Sports Phys Ther 2002;32(1):16–23.

[15] Irrgang JJ, Anderson AF. Development and validation of health-related quality of life measures for the knee. Clin Orthop Relat Res 2002;402:95–109.

[16] Deyo RA. Using outcomes to improve quality of research and quality of care. J Am Board Fam Pract 1998;11(6):465–73.

[17] Osoba D. Lessons learned from measuring health-related quality of life in oncology. J Clin Oncol 1994;12(3):608–16.

[18] Tanner SM, Dainty KN, Marx RG, et al. Knee-specific quality-of-life instruments: Which ones measure symptoms and disabilities most important to patients? Am J Sports Med 2007;35(9):1450–8.

[19] Guyatt GH, Ferrans CE, Halyard MY, et al. Exploration of the value of health-related quality-of-life information from clinical research and into clinical practice. Mayo Clin Proc 2007;82(10):1229–39.

[20] Wilson IB, Cleary PD. Linking clinical variables with health-related quality of life. A conceptual model of patient outcomes. JAMA 1995;273(1):59–65.

[21] Whiteneck G. Conceptual models of disability: past, present, and future. Workshop on disability in America: a new look. Washington, DC: The National Academies Press; 2006.

[22] Jette AM. Physical disablement concepts for physical therapy research and practice. Phys Ther 1994;74(5):380–6.

[23] Nagi S. Some conceptual issues in disability and rehabilitation. In: Sussman M, editor. Sociology and rehabilitation. Washington, DC: American Sociological Association; 1965. p. 100–13.

[24] World Health Organization. ICF—English. Available at: http://www3.who.int/icf/online browser/icf.cfm. Accessed November 22, 2006.

[25] World Health Organization. ICF introduction. Available at: http://www3.who.int/icf/intros/ICF-Eng-Intro.pdf. Accessed October 20, 2006.

[26] Quinn L, Gordon J. Functional outcomes documentation for rehabilitation. St. Louis (MO): W.B. Saunders Company; 2003.

[27] World Health Organization. Towards a common language for functioning, disability and health: ICF. Geneva (IL): World Health Organization; 2002.

[28] Board on Health Science Policy—IOM. The future of disability in America. Washington, DC: The National Academies Press; 2007.

[29] Threats TT. Towards an international framework for communication disorders: use of the ICF. J Commun Disord 2006;39(4):251–65.

[30] Jette AM. The changing language of disablement. Phys Ther 2005;85(2):118–9.

[31] Jette AM. Toward a common language for function, disability, and health. Phys Ther 2006;86(5):726–34.

[32] Levack W. The international classification of functioning, disability, and health (ICF)—application to physiotherapy. New Zealand Journal of Physiotherapy 2004;32(1):1–2.

[33] Hudak PL, Amadio PC, Bombardier C. Development of an upper extremity outcome measure: the DASH (Disabilities of the Arm, Shoulder and Hand). The Upper Extremity Collaborative Group (UECG) [corrected]. Am J Ind Med 1996;29(6):602–8.

[34] Williams GN, Gangel TJ, Arciero RA, et al. Comparison of the single assessment numeric evaluation method and two shoulder rating scales. Outcomes measures after shoulder surgery. Am J Sports Med 1999;27(2):214–21.

[35] Gabel CP, Michener LA, Burkett B, et al. The upper limb functional index: development and determination of reliability, validity, and responsiveness. J Hand Ther 2006;19(3):328–48 [quiz: 349].

[36] Guyatt G, Walter S, Norman G. Measuring change over time: assessing the usefulness of evaluative instruments. J Chronic Dis 1987;40(2):171–8.

[37] Nunnally JC, Bernstein IH. Psychometric theory. New York: McGraw-Hill; 1994.

[38] Portney LG, Watkins MP. Foundations of clinical research: applications to practice. 2nd edition. Upper Saddle River (NJ): Prentice Hall Health; 2000.

[39] Cronbach LJ. Coefficient alpha and the internal structure of tests. Psychometrika 1951;16: 297–334.

[40] Brinker MR, Cuomo JS, Popham GJ, et al. An examination of bias in shoulder scoring instruments among healthy collegiate and recreational athletes. J Shoulder Elbow Surg 2002;11(5):463–9.

[41] Soldatis JJ, Moseley JB, Etminan M. Shoulder symptoms in healthy athletes: a comparison of outcome scoring systems. J Shoulder Elbow Surg 1997;6(3):265–71.

[42] Ware JE Jr, Sherbourne CD. The MOS 36-item short-form health survey (SF-36). I. Conceptual framework and item selection. Med Care 1992;30(6):473–83.

[43] Ware JE Jr, Snow KK, Kosinski M, et al. SF-36 health survey manual and interpretation guide. Boston: The Health Institute; 1993.

[44] McHorney CA, Ware JE Jr, Lu JF, et al. The MOS 36-item Short-Form Health Survey (SF-36): III. Tests of data quality, scaling assumptions, and reliability across diverse patient groups. Med Care 1994;32(1):40–66.

[45] Beaton DE, Katz JN, Fossel AH, et al. Measuring the whole or the parts? Validity, reliability, and responsiveness of the Disabilities of the Arm, Shoulder and Hand outcome measure in different regions of the upper extremity. J Hand Ther. 2001;14(2):128–46.

[46] Gummesson C, Atroshi I, Ekdahl C. The Disabilities of the Arm, Shoulder and Hand (DASH) outcome questionnaire: longitudinal construct validity and measuring self-rated health change after surgery. BMC Musculoskelet Disord 2003;4:11.

[47] Kirkley A, Griffin S, McLintock H, et al. The development and evaluation of a disease-specific quality of life measurement tool for shoulder instability. The Western Ontario Shoulder Instability Index (WOSI). Am J Sports Med 1998;26(6):764–72.

[48] Marx RG, Bombardier C, Wright JG. What do we know about the reliability and validity of physical examination tests used to examine the upper extremity? J Hand Surg [Am] 1999;24(1):185–93.

[49] Schmitt JS, Di Fabio RP. Reliable change and minimum important difference (MID) proportions facilitated group responsiveness comparisons using individual threshold criteria. J Clin Epidemiol 2004;57(10):1008–18.

[50] Richards RR, An KN, Biglianai LU, et al. A standardized method for the assessment of shoulder function. J Shoulder Elbow Surg 1994;3:347–52.

[51] Beaton DE, Richards RR. Measuring function of the shoulder. A cross-sectional comparison of five questionnaires. J Bone Joint Surg Am 1996;78(6):882–90.

[52] Goldhahn J, Angst F, Drerup S, et al. Lessons learned during the cross-cultural adaptation of the American Shoulder and Elbow Surgeons shoulder form into German. J Shoulder Elbow Surg 2008;17(2):248–54.

[53] Kocher MS, Horan MP, Briggs KK, et al. Reliability, validity, and responsiveness of the American Shoulder and Elbow Surgeons subjective shoulder scale in patients with shoulder instability, rotator cuff disease, and glenohumeral arthritis. J Bone Joint Surg Am 2005;87(9):2006–11.

[54] Michener LA, McClure PW, Sennett BJ. American Shoulder and Elbow Surgeons standardized shoulder assessment form, patient self-report section: reliability, validity, and responsiveness. J Shoulder Elbow Surg 2002;11(6):587–94.

[55] Skutek M, Fremerey RW, Zeichen J, et al. Outcome analysis following open rotator cuff repair. Early effectiveness validated using four different shoulder assessment scales. Arch Orthop Trauma Surg 2000;120(7–8):432–6.

[56] Lippitt SB, Harryman DT II, Matsen FA. A practical tool for evaluation of function: the simple shoulder test. In: Matsen FAFF III, Hawkins RJ, editors. The shoulder: a balance of mobility and stability. Rosemont (IL): American Academy of Orthopaedic Surgery; 1993.

[57] Beaton D, Richards RR. Assessing the reliability and responsiveness of 5 shoulder questionnaires. J Shoulder Elbow Surg 1998;7(6):565–72.

[58] Godfrey J, Hamman R, Lowenstein S, et al. Reliability, validity, and responsiveness of the simple shoulder test: psychometric properties by age and injury type. J Shoulder Elbow Surg 2007;16(3):260–7.

[59] Roddey TS, Olson SL, Cook KF, et al. Comparison of the University of California–Los Angeles shoulder scale and the simple shoulder test with the shoulder pain and disability index: single-administration reliability and validity. Phys Ther 2000;80(8):759–68.

[60] van der Windt DA, van der Heijden GJ, de Winter AF, et al. The responsiveness of the shoulder disability questionnaire. Ann Rheum Dis 1998;57(2):82–7.

[61] de Winter AF, van der Heijden GJ, Scholten RJ, et al. The shoulder disability questionnaire differentiated well between high and low disability levels in patients in primary care, in a cross-sectional study. J Clin Epidemiol 2007;60(11):1156–63.

[62] Paul A, Lewis M, Shadforth MF, et al. A comparison of four shoulder-specific questionnaires in primary care. Ann Rheum Dis 2004;63(10):1293–9.

[63] Van der Heijden GJMG, Leffers P, Bouter LM. Shoulder disability questionnaire: design and responsiveness of a functional status measures. J Clin Epidemiol 2000;53:29–38.

[64] Constant CR, Murley AH. A clinical method of functional assessment of the shoulder. Clin Orthop Relat Res 1987;(214):160–4.

[65] Leggin BG, Michener LA, Shaffer MA, et al. The Penn shoulder score: reliability and validity. J Orthop Sports Phys Ther 2006;36(3):138–51.

[66] MacDermid JC, Solomon P, Law M, et al. Defining the effect and mediators of two knowledge translation strategies designed to alter knowledge, intent and clinical utilization of rehabilitation outcome measures: a study protocol [NCT00298727]. Implement Sci 2006;1:14.

Clin Sports Med 27 (2008) 507–519

CLINICS IN SPORTS MEDICINE

ELSEVIER
SAUNDERS

Principles of Restoring Function and Sensorimotor Control in Patients with Shoulder Dysfunction

Brady L. Tripp, PhD, ATC

Department of Athletic Training, College of Nursing and Health Sciences, Florida International University, University Park, ZEB 250B, 11200 Southwest 8th Street, Miami, FL 33199, USA

A delicate balance between mobility and stability affords the shoulder's functional versatility, from controlling large-magnitude forces in opposing football linemen to the fine motor control of a baseball pitcher. Restoring this delicate balance proves challenging to clinicians treating patients who have shoulder dysfunction. To better understand, evaluate, and treat the complexities facing patients who have shoulder dysfunction, practitioners can embrace the art and science inherent to sports medicine. Both basic and applied science has begun to establish the integral role the sensorimotor system (SMS) plays in shoulder function and dysfunction. Although the understanding of the neurosensory and neuromuscular components of shoulder function continues to evolve, the science describes a dynamic and creative neural system that adapts to its environment and in response to practice and experience. When applied, the principles gained through SMS research open the door for vast creativity and variation in the rehabilitation exercises and programs employed. Although embracing such artistic ingenuity may supplement clinical rehabilitation skills, the techniques appear to stand in stark contrast to the standardized, methodical evidence-based practices that have permeated sports medicine. The principles of evidence-based rehabilitation, however, lay in functional outcome and quality-of-life assessments, patient-centered treatment, and whole-person health care. When integrated clinically, the principles of restoring SMS function act in synergy with those of functional outcome-based practices. This article reviews the basic principles of restoring SMS function and evidence-based outcome assessments and describes their integration into treating patients who have shoulder dysfunction.

PRINCIPLES OF RESTORING SENSORIMOTOR SYSTEM FUNCTION

The shoulder's inherent lack of bony stability underscores the demands placed on the SMS to afford the precise neuromuscular control and joint stability needed

E-mail address: trippb@fiu.edu

for normal function [1,2]. SMS function, however, is hampered significantly by shoulder injury [2,3] and fatigue [1,4–7]. Without intervention, diminished SMS function compromises neuromuscular control and functional stability and often cascades into a cycle of further structural damage, fatigue, and dysfunction.

Evidence-Based Surgery and Rehabilitation

Given its critical role in shoulder function, surprisingly few investigations have examined the effectiveness of interventions to restore SMS function. In fact, there are no definitive reports that identify specific factors that restore shoulder SMS function after injury or surgery. Four studies have included shoulder SMS function as a dependent measure after shoulder surgery [8–11]. Although some propose that SMS function returns to normal levels 2 to 7 years after surgery [8–10], results of others do not [11]. In either case, the ability to draw conclusions from their results is limited by the design and methods employed in each report, including:

- Failure to measure the same patients preoperatively and postoperatively [9–11]
- Failure to provide any structured or supervised rehabilitation program or track patients' progress or participation in rehabilitation [8–11]
- Failure to compare measures to a control group [9,10]

Because many surgical options for treating shoulder dysfunction alter or displace the capsular, muscular, or neural tissues that provide afferent and efferent feedback to the SMS, further research should investigate SMS function after surgery.

During postsurgical rehabilitation and conservative treatment of shoulder dysfunction, clinicians commonly employ dynamic stabilization, joint position sense, and plyometric exercises in hopes of enhancing or restoring SMS function to the shoulder [12,13]. Little empiric evidence, however, describes the effectiveness of such programs. One report suggests that 6 weeks of plyometric training may enhance some specific components of SMS function in healthy shoulders [12], while results after similar programs have failed to support this finding [14]. Although additional research is warranted to identify specific aspects of surgery and rehabilitation that may enhance SMS function in the shoulder, one is able to elicit a few recommendations from the current body of research. Surgery to restore structural integrity of the unstable glenohumeral joint may aid SMS function in the long term and appears advantageous. When appropriate (healthy shoulders or in late rehabilitation), plyometric glenohumeral rotation exercises using elastic tubing and weighted-ball throwing and catching may promote SMS function. In summary, clinicians treating patients who have shoulder dysfunction can draw several implications from this literature that will be highlighted in the following sections, including:

- Lack of research limits evidence-based practices
- Surgically restoring the integrity of unstable shoulders may yield long-term SMS benefits
- Plyometrics may facilitate SMS function in healthy shoulders

Rehabilitation (concepts or exercises) for restoring sensorimotor system function
Without research that clearly identifies factors that restore SMS function, practicing evidence-based rehabilitation for patients who have shoulder dysfunction is challenging. One can draw recommendations, however, from both applied and basic science. Sound research, coupled with growing consensus from clinicians, suggests that stability of the kinetic chain is critical to shoulder function [15,16]. The SMS plays a critical role in control of the kinetic chain through both feedforward and feedback mechanisms. Research suggests that musculoskeletal dysfunction often is associated with deficits in the feedforward mechanism that provide the proximal stability needed for normal distal function [17]. Clinicians treating patients who have shoulder dysfunction thereby are encouraged to evaluate stability from the ground up, from the ankle, knee, and hip through the trunk (core), to the scapulothoracic and glenohumeral joints [18]. Integrating such motions as the single-leg squat, lunges, and step-ups into the evaluation and rehabilitation exercises clearly is warranted.

Functional shoulder stability also is facilitated by promoting the critical force couples of glenohumeral stabilizers. These include closed kinetic chain exercises and employing an axial load to the shoulder [14,19]. Exercises such as weight-shifts, table-slides and wall-slides can be used safely early in rehabilitation programs, because they produce low to moderate rotator cuff activation while avoiding the large shear forces often produced by the deltoids during open-chain exercises [19]. Research using healthy individuals can provide clinicians valuable insight into exercises that target specific core muscles that are critical to proximal shoulder stability, including the lower and middle trapezius and serratus anterior. Isolating specific muscles is appropriate early in rehabilitation to assure activation and endurance. Exercises should move from isolated muscle activity to integrated functional movements as soon as appropriate tissue healing is assured. Both well-established [20] and recent [21,22] reports have identified exercises that optimally activate the key scapulothoracic stabilizers such as the lower and middle trapezius and serratus anterior while avoiding dominance of the upper trapezius. The lower and middle trapezius are activated effectively by side-lying external rotation, side-lying forward flexion, and prone horizontal abduction with external rotation [22]. Prone arm extension also may target the middle trapezius [22] while the serratus anterior is isolated best through push-up exercises [21]. In summary, this literature leads to several implications for treating patients who have shoulder dysfunction:

- Integrate lower-extremity kinetic chain movements into evaluation and rehabilitation (eg, single-leg squat, lunges, and set-ups)
- Initiate upper-extremity closed-chain exercises early in rehabilitation
- Isolate core scapulothoracic muscles using valid exercises
- Transition from muscle isolation to functional movements early in rehabilitation

Evidence-Based Neuromuscular Rehabilitation

Without research-validated programs, one can gain valuable insight into the foundation of the SMS through research emerging from basic neuroscience.

Clinicians clearly understand application of the overload principle (specific adaptation to imposed demands) in rehabilitation to facilitate adaptive changes in muscle tissue. The initial gains in strength programs that are not caused by muscle hypertrophy are traditionally attributed to enhanced neuromuscular efficiency [23]. Recent research into a nervous system once thought to be rigid and resistant to change, suggests that both anatomic and functional changes in neural tissue are able to compensate for damage after injury and also adapt as a result of practice and experience [17,24]. It is clear that understanding the principles governing neuromuscular plasticity can be applied to facilitate changes in SMS function and improve clinical effectiveness [17].

Cutting-edge neuroscience and motor-control research using functional MRI, motor-evoked potentials, and transcranial magnetic potentials is shedding light on the mechanisms by which our SMS learns, adapts and develops motor programs. Research suggests that learning-induced neuroplasticity can be positive or negative, and structural and functional at the highest level. Even the highest levels of the nervous system will alter their anatomy to compensate for injured tissue and accomplish directed goals [25]. Comparing athletes from different sports, researchers observed differences in cortical representations of muscles and movements [26]. Volleyball athletes displayed larger cortical maps for control of shoulder muscles when compared with runners [26]. Their findings suggest that the specific sport/activity drove neuroplasticity at the highest level. Research observing novice jugglers suggests that learning a new, complex, dynamic task that requires precise neuromuscular control results in anatomic and functional changes to the motor cortex [27]. Interestingly, when participants refrained from juggling for 9 weeks, all changes to the motor cortex reverted just as quickly as they formed [27]. Additional evidence also suggests that more complex and intellectually challenging motor skills are more effective in driving neuroplasticity [28]. The authors noted, however, that there is variability between an individual patient's perception of task difficulty, and thus choosing extremely difficult tasks may be counterproductive. It appears clear that neural tissue can adapt anatomically and functionally to injury, practice, and task difficulty; however, changes are lost quickly if new motor programs are abandoned. Applying these principles, clinicians should be aware that negative, compensatory motor programs might already be engrained when they initially evaluate a patient. Clinicians can encourage development of positive motor programs by having patients practice beneficial movements they wish to instill soon after injury or surgery. Patients can be proactive and practice positive motor programs preoperatively or before using supportive devices such as slings and braces. Clinicians should prescribe movements the patient can practice regularly throughout the course of his or her day to replace or avoid compensatory motor programs. Prescribing tasks that require complex and novel movements is encouraged. It is also important to recognize that new motor programs decay when unused, and clinicians should reassess functional motor programs regularly throughout rehabilitation.

Researchers also are learning that neuromuscular plasticity is task-specific and that motor programs developed by practicing only part of a movement may not carryover to the whole task [17]. The clinical implications of this finding to rehabilitation are clear and easily put into practice. Exercises that isolate specific muscles should be used early in rehabilitation, but sparingly. Therapeutic exercises should transition to functional motions early. Additional research indicates that development of new motor programs is facilitated by practicing systematic and progressive variations of the task. Varying task demands such as the body position, along with the magnitude, speed, and direction of movement and applied resistance will create a more robust, efficient, and functional motor program [29]. Clinicians can apply these principles directly by practicing whole, functional movements as early as possible in rehabilitation. It seems that employing creativity and artistic ingenuity to progressively vary functional exercises will capitalize on neuroplasticity. Recognizing the litany of variables that clinicians can choose to manipulate illustrates the broad range of possible functional task variations (Table 1). Although the precise number of repetitions needed to develop or change motor plans remains unclear, clinicians should consider the number of times a negative motor program may be practiced in the course of a patient's day. It is clear that engraining motor programs may require well more than the 15 to 45 repetitions traditionally prescribed. As research continues to uncover the potential of neuroplasticity, it will certainly add significantly to clinical practice. In summary, this body of literature leads to several implications for treating patients who have shoulder dysfunction:

- Proactive training may help avoid compensatory motor programs
- Employ complex, physically and intellectually challenging tasks
- Engrain effective motor programs using activities that can be repeated throughout the day
- Use progressive variation of activities to develop robust motor programs
- Reassess functional motor programs regularly throughout rehabilitation

PRINCIPLES OF USING PATIENT-CENTERED TREATMENT AND FUNCTIONAL OUTCOME ASSESSMENTS

To enhance the quality of health care provided, one must systematically evaluate the effectiveness of clinical treatments for patients who have shoulder dysfunction by employing and contributing to evidence-based practices. Functional outcome assessments such as the DASH (disabilities of the arm, shoulder and hand) [30], the SST (simple shoulder test) [31], the WOSI (Western Ontario Shoulder Instability Index) [32], and the WORC (Western Ontario Rotator Cuff Index) [33] provide clinicians with reliable and objective measures of each patient's shoulder function to document progress and compare with established norms. Ideally, clinicians employ tools designed and validated for use with their specific patient population. Currently, however, few shoulder-specific functional outcome assessments have been validated for use with athletes. Tools that include athlete-specific components include the DASH sports module [30] and the Athletic Shoulder Outcome Scoring System [34]. Common components of these tools include assessments of range of motion, pain, and

Table 1
Variables that clinicians can manipulate throughout rehabilitation to progress functional tasks and create robust, efficient motor programs

Variable	Activity progression
Integrated joint motion	Lower-extremity and trunk → scapula → glenohumeral → elbow → entire-extremity
Muscle activity	Isolated isometrics → reactive isometrics → isolated isotonic → integrated functional motion (isotonic) → plyometric
Kinetic chain	Closed → open → variable
Plane of motion	Single-plane → multi-plane
Resistance lever arm	Short → long → variable
Resistance applied	Single-plane → multiplane
Resistance direction	Axial load → variable
Resistance intensity	Low → high → variable
Task speed	Slow → fast → variable
Environment	Stable → unstable → variable
Visual input	Eyes open → eyes closed
Tactile input	Protective device → manual → none

the ability of the athlete to perform ADLs and return to his or her preinjury level of sport activity. Instruments such as these reflect the specific aim of clinicians in sports medicine, to return athletes to their preinjury level of sport/activity; therefore they will remain critical components of our practice. Relying on such tools to judge clinical success, however, may assume that an athlete's quality of life has been restored upon his or her return to sport/activity. This assumption is often misleading, prompting suggestions that relying solely on such focused tools will limit the progress of enhancing clinical practices [35,36]. Clinicians should use two functional outcome assessments when treating patients who have shoulder dysfunction (1) a shoulder-specific functional outcome tool that quantifies a return-to-activity level that is appropriate for their patient-population and (2) an integrated, whole-person tool that assesses function and disability.

Growing international consensus favors a universal, whole-person, patient-centered, and multidisciplinary team approach to assessing and treating function and disability. Particularly in orthopedics, quality of life and measures of functional ability will soon become the benchmarks against which clinicians will examine the effectiveness of treatments [34]. The most widely-accepted measure of one's functional ability is the International Classification of Functioning, Disability, and Health (ICF) [37]. Published in 2001, the ICF illustrates a complex integration of the whole patient and his or her environment that includes body functions and structures and personal and environmental factors (psychology, pain management, coping strategies, and medicinal interventions) [37]. Although reviewing the processes of using the ICF to guide evaluation and rehabilitation is beyond the scope of this article, many comprehensive reviews are available [36,38]. The ICF employs a multidisciplinary team approach to examine and treat the patient's impairment in the context of his or her activity and participation in his or her environment. A critical goal of any patient-centered approach is to make the patient an active participant in the evaluation and treatment process. This begins with using a standard patient-rated questionnaire that includes the patient's subjective description of his or her functional limitations. Treating athletes, one often assumes their goal is to return to play. Using a patient-centered tool, however, will help distinguish between the perspectives of the patient, clinician, and others included in the rehabilitation team (eg, coach, orthopedic surgeon, psychologist). After reviewing the patient's completed questionnaire, the clinician performs an orthopedic evaluation to identify anatomic or functional problems in body function that are limiting the patient's activity or participation. This includes standard clinical assessments of neurovascular function, posture, strength, flexibility, endurance, neuromuscular control, and joint stability. After all assessments are complete, the team identifies the functional limitations using the patient's own words and relates each functional limitation to relevant and modifiable factors. For example, the patient may identify the inability to sleep through the night as a limitation following shoulder surgery. Each member of the team may identify contributing factors:

- The team physician identifies local inflammation and a lack of appropriate medication.
- The clinician identifies poor shoulder strength and flexibility.
- The psychologist identifies poor living conditions and social factors.

The team then identifies patient-driven functional goals (eg, sleeping through the night without pain) and factors to address (enhance shoulder strength and flexibility). With athletes, functional goals should include quality-of-life and sport-specific goals, particularly early in rehabilitation. Failing to specify easily achievable patient-driven goals such as self-care, independent mobility, or a recreational skill may affect the athlete's quality of life significantly and limit clinical effectiveness in turn. The final staple of the patient-centered whole-person approach is to assess and record the patient's progress systematically using the same multidisciplinary evaluation techniques. Clinicians should include the appropriate shoulder-specific functional outcome tool and measure of function and disability used initially. In summary, this literature leads to several implications for treating patients with shoulder dysfunction:

- Evaluate and treat the patient as a whole person; make the patient an active participant
- Use a multidisciplinary team approach and a patient-rated quality-of-life questionnaire
- Include a shoulder-specific functional outcome tool and standardized clinical measures
- Set patient-driven functional goals that require the foundations for the patient's activity
- Systematically assess each patient's progress and function

PRINCIPLES OF INTEGRATED REHABILITATION FOR PATIENTS WHO HAVE SHOULDER DYSFUNCTION

1. Evaluate and treat the patient as a whole-person; make patient an active participant in the process. Use a multidisciplinary approach and a standard patient-rated quality-of-life questionnaire. Include a shoulder-specific functional outcome tool and standardized clinical measures.
2. Use patient's descriptions to identify functional limitations; identify limiting factors.
3. Set patient-driven, functional goals that require the foundations for the patient's activity.
4. Recognize and capitalize on neuromuscular plasticity throughout rehabilitation. Interrupt compensatory motor programs; engrain functional, robust motor programs.
5. Practice whole, functional patient-driven activities early and often.
6. Stress proximal stability; it is the foundation of function. Integrate lower-extremity kinetic chain movements into evaluation and rehabilitation. Build the foundation early (trunk and scapular control) through postural awareness and closed-chain exercises before progressing distally. Engrain motor programs that begin with proximal stability, include scapular setting.
7. Use progressive variation of tasks to address all rehabilitation goals. Use complex and intellectually engaging tasks.
8. Include routine assessments of progress and function. Use a patient-rated quality-of-life questionnaire, a shoulder-specific functional outcome tool and standardized clinical measures.

PRINCIPLES IN PRACTICE

Integrating the principles of restoring SMS function with a patient-centered, quality-of-life paradigm provides a dynamic, creative, robust framework for treating patients who have shoulder dysfunction. Practicing these principles frees the clinician to explore a broad range of variations on functional, patient-driven activities while still employing evidence-based methods. Although patient-driven goals are individualized, the foundations of sound shoulder function are constant. Examples of functional goals for three broad phases of rehabilitation are presented along with task progressions to achieve each goal.

Early Rehabilitation

Goals chosen for early rehabilitation should include tasks that require the basic foundations for the patient's functional activity. Such goals may be to complete an activity that requires any or all foundations of shoulder function including pain control, soft tissue and basic joint mobility, basic muscle activation, postural correction and awareness, and trunk and scapular stability and control. Patients can strive to achieve many of these goals preoperatively as well, by introducing and practicing effective motor programs while wearing the protective device (eg, sling or brace) that the patient will wear after surgery. Typical goals would be activities requiring the patient to attain scapular postural awareness and neuromuscular control by finding and stabilizing the scapular set position in retraction and depression. The ideal scapular set position that is vital to shoulder stability is difficult to achieve and maintain without flexible anterior (pectoralis major and minor) and posterior (capsule and external rotators) structures, strength, endurance and control of the core scapular stabilizing muscles, and adequate thoracic extension. A patient-driven goal may be the patient brushing his or her teeth and hair comfortably. The patient must progress in each foundation to achieve this goal (adequate pain control, flexibility, strength, endurance, postural awareness, and scapular control). Other foundational goals, chosen preoperatively or during early rehabilitation may be to progress through a series of variations on the scapular clock and shoulder dump exercise to promote postural and scapular awareness and control while wearing a sling (Fig. 1).

Recovery Phase

Foundational goals for the recovery phases of rehabilitation include activities that require full range of motion, up to 75% of strength and endurance, good static and dynamic proximal stability (lower-extremity, trunk, scapula), and progress from static to dynamic glenohumeral joint stability. Tasks usually begin with challenging isometric stability. A foundational goal for the recovery phase may be to complete a rhythmic stabilization series of both closed- and open-chain tasks progressing from table to wall with variations in the plane, speed, and intensity of direction, performed with eyes open and closed. The tasks progress to facilitate range of motion and dynamic stability from table slides through diagonal wall slides and end with open-chain lawnmower exercises (Fig. 2).

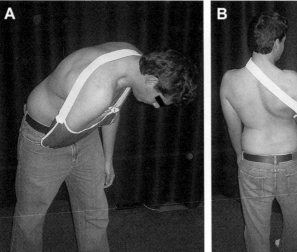

Fig. 1. A step-initiated shoulder dump (A, B) integrates the lower-extremity and core, encourages thoracic extension and scapular retraction and depression on return.

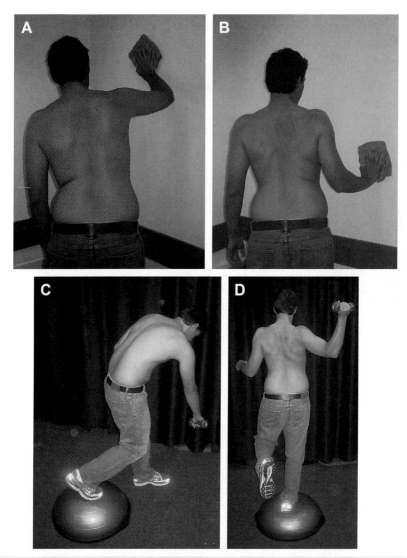

Fig. 2. Diagonal wall-slides (*A, B*) facilitate range of motion, lower trapezius and serratus anterior activation, and neuromuscular control; shoulder dumps progress to step-back lawn-mower exercises (*C, D*) to achieve dynamic stability in a functional position.

Late Phase

Foundational goals for the late phase of rehabilitation should progress to activities that require functional levels of power, endurance, neuromuscular control, and full kinetic chain motions. Patient-driven functional activities should progress through multiple combinations and manipulations of each appropriate variable (Table 1). Tasks should aim to develop robust, functional motor programs that can adapt to unforeseen obstacles and abrupt manipulation of each appropriate variable. A football lineman or wrestler must progress to the functional activity of blocking or controlling an opponent, a task requiring the shoulder to play a vital role as part of the kinetic chain. In a difficult and endurance-testing environment, the athlete must respond to and control a resistance that has extreme variability in its speed, intensity, and direction. A goal may begin with a push-up progression through various levels of stability, muscle contraction, speed, and planes, and moves from tabletop to wall to the floor before progressing to step-up-and-overs and other challenging plyometrics and medicine ball tosses (Fig. 3).

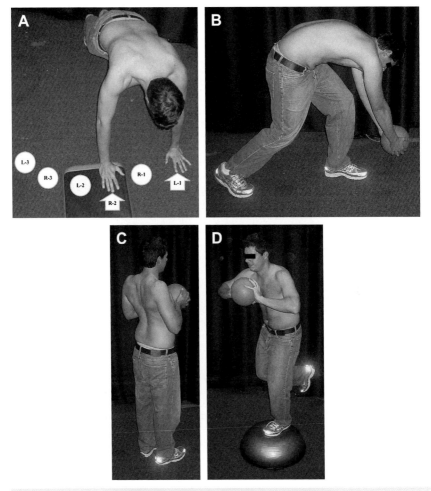

Fig. 3. A push-up and medicine ball progression includes a timed series of step-up-and-overs (A), lunges (B, C), and step-up chest passes (D). (A) Circles indicate the order of (R) right and (L) left hand positions; arrows indicate current hand position.

SUMMARY

When integrated clinically, outcome-based practices act in synergy to create dynamic and robust guidelines to treating patients who have shoulder dysfunction. Clinicians should consider regular use of appropriate outcome assessments and following a whole-person treatment and assessment paradigm. Exercises should include practicing whole, functional, patient-driven activities that require the foundations of sound shoulder function and include the entire kinetic chain. Clinicians can capitalize on neuromuscular plasticity by incorporating progressive variation of functional activities to engrain robust, effective motor programs early and often throughout rehabilitation.

References

[1] Myers JB, Lephart SM. Sensorimotor deficits contributing to glenohumeral instability. Clin Orthop Relat Res 2002;400:98–104.

[2] Myers JB, Lephart SM. The role of the sensorimotor system in the athletic shoulder. J Athl Train 2000;35(3):351–63.

[3] Borsa PA, Lephart SM, Kocher MS, et al. Functional assessment and rehabilitation of shoulder proprioception for glenohumeral instability. J Sport Rehabil 1994;3(1):84–104.

[4] Allen TJ, Proske U. Effect of muscle fatigue on the sense of limb position and movement. Exp Brain Res 2006;170(1):30–8.

[5] Carpenter JE, Blasier RB, Pellizzon GG. The effects of muscle fatigue on shoulder joint position sense. Am J Sports Med 1998;26(2):262–5.

[6] Tripp BL, Boswell L, Gansneder BM, et al. Functional fatigue decreases 3-dimensional multijoint position reproduction acuity in the overhead-throwing athlete. J Athl Train 2004;39(4):316–20.

[7] Tripp BL, Uhl TL, Yochem EM. Functional fatigue decreases upper-extremity sensorimotor system acuity in baseball athletes. J Athl Train 2007;42(1):90–8.

[8] Potzl W, Thorwesten L, Gotze C, et al. Proprioception of the shoulder joint after surgical repair for instability: a long-term follow-up study. Am J Sports Med 2004;32(2):425–30.

[9] Aydin T, Yildiz Y, Yanmis I, et al. Shoulder proprioception: a comparison between the shoulder joint in healthy and surgically repaired shoulders. Arch Orthop Trauma Surg 2001;121(7):422–5.

[10] Lephart SM, Myers JB, Bradley JP, et al. Shoulder proprioception and function following thermal capsulorraphy. Arthroscopy 2002;18(7):770–8.

[11] Fremerey R, Bosch U, Lobenhoffer P, et al. Joint position awareness and sports activity after capsulolabral reconstruction in the overhead athlete. Int J Sports Med 2006;27(8):648–52.

[12] Swanik KA, Lephart SM, Swanik CB, et al. The effects of shoulder plyometric training on proprioception and selected muscle performance characteristics. J Shoulder Elbow Surg 2002;11(6):579–86.

[13] Wilk KE, Reinold MM, Andrews JR. Rehabilitation of the thrower's elbow. Clin Sports Med 2004;23(4):765–801.

[14] Padua DA, Guskiewicz KM, Prentice WE, et al. The effect of select shoulder exercises on strength, active angle reproduction, single-arm balance, and functional performance. J Sport Rehabil 2004;13(1):75–95.

[15] Broer MR. Efficiency of human movement. 3rd edition. Philadelphia: W.B. Saunders Co.; 1973.

[16] Kibler WB. Closed kinetic chain rehabilitation for sports injuries. Phys Med Rehabil Clin N Am 2000;11(2):369–84.

[17] van Vliet PM, Heneghan NR. Motor control and the management of musculoskeletal dysfunction. Man Ther 2006;11(3):208–13.

[18] Kibler WB, McMullen J, Uhl T. Shoulder rehabilitation strategies, guidelines, and practice. Orthop Clin North Am 2001;32(3):527–38.

[19] Uhl TL, Carver TJ, Mattacola CG, et al. Shoulder musculature activation during upper extremity weight-bearing exercise. J Orthop Sports Phys Ther 2003;33(3):109–17.

[20] Moseley JB Jr, Jobe FW, Pink M, et al. EMG analysis of the scapular muscles during a shoulder rehabilitation program. Am J Sports Med 1992;20(2):128–34.

[21] Ludewig PM, Hoff MS, Osowski EE, et al. Relative balance of serratus anterior and upper trapezius muscle activity during push-up exercises. Am J Sports Med 2004;32(2):484–93.

[22] Cools AM, Dewitte V, Lanszweert F, et al. Rehabilitation of scapular muscle balance: which exercises to prescribe? Am J Sports Med 2007;35(10):1744–51.

[23] Sale DG. Neural adaptation to resistance training. Med Sci Sports Exerc 1988;20(5): S135–45.

[24] Kelly C, Foxe JJ, Garavan H. Patterns of normal human brain plasticity after practice and their implications for neurorehabilitation. Arch Phys Med Rehabil 2006;87(12 Suppl 2): S20–9.

[25] Robertson IH, Murre JMJ. Rehabilitation of brain damage: brain plasticity and principles of guided recovery. Psychol Bull 1999;125(5):544–75.

[26] Tyc F, Boyadjian A, Devanne H. Motor cortex plasticity induced by extensive training revealed by transcranial magnetic stimulation in human. Eur J Neurosci 2005;21(1): 259–66.

[27] Draganski B, Gaser C, Busch V, et al. Neuroplasticity: changes in grey matter induced by training. Nature 2004;427(6972):311–2.

[28] Carey JR, Bhatt E, Nagpal A. Neuroplasticity promoted by task complexity. Exerc Sport Sci Rev 2005;33(1):24–31.

[29] Dean CM, Shepherd RB. Task-related training improves performance of seated reaching tasks after stroke. A randomized controlled trial. Stroke 1997;28(4):722–8.

[30] Hudak PL, Amadio PC, Bombardier C. Development of an upper extremity outcome measure: the DASH (disabilities of the arm, shoulder and hand) [corrected]. The upper extremity collaborative group (UECG). Am J Ind Med 1996;29(6):602–8.

[31] Lippitt SB, Harryman DT, Matsen FA. A practical tool for evaluating function: the simple shoulder test. In: The shoulder: a balance of mobility and stability. Rosemont (IL): American Academy of Orthopaedic Surgeons; 1993. p. 501–18.

[32] Kirkley A, Griffin S, McLintock H, et al. The development and evaluation of a disease-specific quality of life measurement tool for shoulder instability. The western Ontario shoulder instability index (WOSI). Am J Sports Med 1998;26(6):764–72.

[33] Kirkley A, Alvarez C, Griffin S. The development and evaluation of a disease-specific quality-of-life questionnaire for disorders of the rotator cuff: the Western Ontario Rotator Cuff Index. Clin J Sport Med 2003;13(2):84–92.

[34] Matsen FA III, Smith KL, DeBartolo SE, et al. A comparison of patients with late-stage rheumatoid arthritis and osteoarthritis of the shoulder using self-assessed shoulder function and health status. Arthritis Care Res 1997;10:43–7.

[35] Meller R, Krettek C, Gosling T, et al. Recurrent shoulder instability among athletes: changes in quality of life, sports activity, and muscle function following open repair. Knee Surg Sports Traumatol Arthrosc 2007;15(3):295–304.

[36] Steiner WA, Ryser L, Huber E, et al. Use of the ICF model as a clinical problem-solving tool in physical therapy and rehabilitation medicine. Phys Ther 2002;82(11):1098–107.

[37] World Health Organization. International classification of functioning, disability, and health (ICF) ICF full version ed. Geneva (Switzerland): World Health Organization; 2001.

[38] Jette AM. Toward a common language for function, disability, and health. Phys Ther 2006;86(5):726–34.

Clin Sports Med 27 (2008) 521–526

CLINICS IN SPORTS MEDICINE

INDEX

A

Alpha motor neuron, afferent, 483

Anesthetics, local, to reverse arthrogenic muscle inhibition, 413–414

Ankle, chronic instability of, and ankle sprains, sensorimotor deficits with, **353–370**
    inversion perturbation in, 358
    measures of jump landings in, 362–363
    motoneuron pool excitability in, 357–358
    of acute ankle sprain, gait in, 362
    outcomes of, balance/coordination training and, 376–377
    postural control in, 360–361
    proprioception in, 356–357
    strength deficits in, 359
injury of, external support after, future directions in, 374–375
instability of, and sensorimotor deficits, contemporary theory of, 363–365
    continuum of, 377–379
    external support in, 377–378
    sensorimotor deficits and, 365
    traditional theory of, and sensorimotor deficits, 354–356
sprains of, acute, deficit in isometric strength in, 359
    or chronic ankle instability, gait in, 362
    postural control in, 360
    proprioception in, 356
    acute lateral, outcomes of, balance/coordination training and, 376
    and chronic ankle instability, sensorimotor deficits with, **353–370**
    balance/coordination training and, future directions in, 377
    first time and recurrent, interventions for prevention of, **371–382**
    inversion perturbation in, 358
    lateral, outcomes of, external support and, 373–374
    ligamentous injury in, 353
    prevalence of, in high school students, 371
    prevention of, 372
        balance/coordination training and, 375–377
        external support and, 372–375
    risk factors associated with, 371–372
    stability of, muscle strength and, 358–359

Anterior cruciate ligament, composition of, 383
    damaged, gamma motor neuron dysfunction in, 388
    injury of, assessment of function following, 395–396
        biomechanical compensatory changes in, 392–395
        gait following, 393–394
        hamstring muscle torque following, 390
        hypothesis concerning, 386
        in female athletes, body core and lower extremity alignments and, 427
            growth and maturation and, 426–427
            increased risk of, biomechanics related to, 426
            neuromuscular training in reduction of, 426
            risk of, factors increasing, 425–426, 427, 428
        jogging/running electromyography in, 394
        jogging/running following, 394
        jogging/running kinematics following, 394
        jogging/running kinetics following, 394
        muscle activation in, 385–386

Note: Page numbers of article titles are in **boldface** type.

0278-5919/08/$ – see front matter
doi:10.1016/S0278-5919(08)00037-9

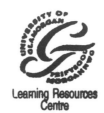

Learning Resources
Centre